The Physician's Assistant

Ann Suter Ford

The Physician's Assistant

A National and Local Analysis

PRAEGER SPECIAL STUDIES IN U.S. ECONOMIC, SOCIAL, AND POLITICAL ISSUES

Praeger Publishers New York Washington London

Library of Congress Cataloging in Publication Data

Ford, Ann Suter.
The physician's assistant.

(Praeger special studies in U.S. economic, social, and political issues)
Bibliography: p.
1. Physicians' assistants--United States.
I. Title. [DNLM: 1. Physicians' assistants.
W21.5 F699p] Nov. 11, 1975
R697.P45F67 1975 610.69'53'0973 73-8391
ISBN 0-275-28855-2

PRAEGER PUBLISHERS
111 Fourth Avenue, New York, N.Y. 10003, U.S.A.
5, Cromwell Place, London SW7 2JL, England

Published in the United States of America in 1975
by Praeger Publishers, Inc.

Printed in the United States of America

For my parents and
for Scott and Tracey

PREFACE

This book investigates the development of a new health professional: the physician's assistant. Designed as an exploratory study, it attempts to incorporate theory and empirical findings in order to promote a better understanding of the problems encountered by innovators in the health field. Theoretical insights are borrowed from several traditions: diffusion of innovations, resistance to change, social and organizational conflict, and health manpower. Existing literature on the physician's assistant is integrated with the author's own survey data. The survey data were the result of three separate studies: two national surveys of early physician's assistant programs at two different time periods and one local case study. The book concludes with a brief discussion of the broader implications of such research both for the immediate subject under study (the physician's assistant) and for the broader area of health manpower innovations.

This study began as a master's thesis, although in its present form it is substantially expanded and revised to give it broader applicability. Many of the findings of this research are presently being incorporated by the author into a doctoral dissertation devoted to an examination of the physician's assistant vis-a-vis the nurse practitioner from the perspectives of both the programs and their practicing graduates.

The author gratefully acknowledges the considerable time and interest given this research by the survey respondents: the PA and NP program directors in the national surveys and the physicians, nurses, and patients participating in the local study. Without their sustained interest, obviously, there could have been no study. Financial support for part of the research was provided by the Department of Urban and Regional Planning and the Urban Research Center, Institute for Social Research, The Florida State University, Tallahassee. A special acknowledgement is reserved for Professors Robert Ollry and Edward E. McClure for their continuing interest in the research effort. Finally, and most importantly, the author gratefully acknowledges the patience, the encouragement, and the considerable help given her throughout the entire research project by her husband, W. Scott Ford.

CONTENTS

LIST OF TABLES AND FIGURES

LIST OF ABBREVIATIONS

AAP	American Academy of Pediatrics
AHA	American Hospital Association
AMA	American Medical Association
ANA	American Nurses' Association
APHA	American Public Health Association
CA	Clinical Associate
FNP	Family Nurse Practitioner
HMO	Health Maintenance Organization
LPN	Licensed Practical Nurse
MNA	Medical Nurse Associate
NA	Nurse Associate
NAS	National Academy of Sciences
NLN	National League for Nursing
NP	Nurse Practitioner
PA	Physician's Assistant
PNP/PNA	Pediatric Nurse Practitioner/Pediatric Nurse Associate
RN	Registered Nurse

The Physician's Assistant

CHAPTER

1

THE EMERGENCE OF A NEW HEALTH PROFESSIONAL

INTRODUCTION

With the emergence of a new social consciousness in the United States during the 1960s, accessible quality health care was asserted by many to be a right and not a privilege of all citizens. Although an admirable long-range goal to guide the development of health policy, was it a realistic one? Critics both from outside and from within the major health professions began to question the ability of the present system to meet this new challenge. As segments of the health delivery system were subjected to analysis, inadequacies were identified. One such inadequacy was the apparent gap between the growing and anticipated demand for health care and the potential supply of health providers to deliver the required services.

Many factors have contributed to what some have termed a crisis situation in the health manpower area. Rising incomes are allowing more people to effectively demand access to increased quality and quantity of health services. A generally rising level of education has made more people aware of their need for health care; education affects not only one's definition of health but also influences how effectively one can utilize the health system to satisfy his needs. Technological and biomedical advances have contributed to the efficacy of the health care provided thus promoting a greater desire to consume the services. The increased involvement of government in the financing of health care for the aged (Medicare) and the poor (Medicaid) have increased the power of these often medically disenfranchised groups to demand better health care. In addition, expansion of private third-party health plans for basic coverage has encouraged many people to expend significant portions of their discretionary income for health care. With the very real possibility of some type of national health insurance becoming operational in the mid to late 1970s, the demands for health services will be increasingly felt. Fein has estimated that an expanding population base and changing age-sex distribution coupled with rising levels of income and education as well as the effect of governmental third-party payments will increase the demand for physician services between 1965 and 1975 by between 22 percent and 26 percent. This projected increase in demand is "an estimate of the amount consumers, given their 1975 demographic and socioeconomic characteristics would be prepared to purchase at today's [1967] relative prices."[1]

In order to accommodate the anticipated increase in demand, many changes in the delivery of health services must be instituted. One of these changes will involve policies relating to augmenting the supply of existing health professionals. Although such augmentation may be accomplished in several ways, two approaches have received the most attention: (1) increase the supply of existing health professionals; and (2) increase the productivity of existing health providers. Acknowledging that neither approach is likely to be the solution nor that the two approaches are exclusionary, which approach seems most likely to yield the desired results given an acceptable period of adjustment?

V. R. Fuchs has estimated that the average cost of educating a physician is greater than $1000, 000.[2] However, Chris Theodore has aptly noted that when considering the cost of additional medical manpower vis-a-vis other types of health providers, it is "only the marginal cost of production, namely the cost of educating an additional medical graduate. . ." which should be considered.[3] This position would argue for increasing our supply of medical graduates by utilizing existing medical schools more efficiently; for example, shortening the medical school curriculum from four to three years. Citing the heavy initial capital outlay, and continuing operational expenses of creating just one new medical school as well as the time lag between initiation of a new school and the appearance of the first graduate (seven years), the additional years required for internship and residency (three years), and the debt caused by withdrawing active practitioners to provide faculty (five years), Harvey Estes has noted the advantages accruing to increasing the output of existing medical schools as opposed to developing new schools.[4]

Both Theodore and Estes would acknowledge that a substantial increase in the production of physicians is a valid long range goal. The health manpower shortage, however, is a problem of immediate importance. In addition, many have concluded that much of the health manpower problem is one of productivity and maldistribution as opposed to being a primarily numerical one.[5] Fein has noted that even a "three percent increase in productivity could increase the effective supply of physicians by the equivalent of one year's graduating class."[6]

How can such increases in productivity be achieved? Several means have been suggested: improvements in organizational patterns; changes in delivery systems; the use of computers and other means of automating the provision of health care; and the introduction of new types of health providers to augment and assist the activities of existing health professionals who are in short supply. It is an examination of this latter approach to increasing productivity that provides the focus for the present study; that is, this book is devoted to a study of a new type of health provider: the physician's assistant (PA).

THE PHYSICIAN'S ASSISTANT

The physician's assistant, a newcomer to the health field, was the focus of a 1970 report of the Board on Medicine of the National Academy of Sciences (NAS).[7] The Report divided the broader concept of the PA into three more succinct levels or categories of personnel:

1. The physician's associate (Type A). This individual is the most highly trained type of assistant. He would be capable of assisting the physician by performing diagnostic and therapeutic procedures and coordinating the roles of other, more technical, assistants. While he would function under the general supervision and responsibility of the physician, he might, under special circumstances, perform without the immediate surveillance of the physician. He may be expected to exercise a degree of independent medical judgment.

2. The specialist assistant (Type B). This individual is highly skilled in one type of clinical specialty or procedures within a specialty. Although he has a limited area of knowledge and skill, he has a depth of training and skill within this area which is exceeded only by the specialist-physician working within the same field. He is less capable of independent action than the physician's associate.

3. The nonspecialized assistant (Type C). This individual would be capable of performing a variety of tasks over the whole range of medical care under the supervision of a physician with whom this assistant would work in close proximity. He does not have the level of knowledge necessary to integrate and interpret the findings he has obtained in his testing of the patient. Generally his training is less formal than that of either the physician's associate or specialized assistant; much of his training is obtained by on-the-job experience with the physician for whom he will work.[8]

Since the present book was an attempt to examine the overall status and acceptability of this new health professional, a broad generic interpretation of the concept was adopted. Thus, while acknowledging the utility of a more refined delineation of types of PAs, this research classified all three NAS categories as physician's assistants.

Although the first PA program began in 1965, by 1970 many fundamental issues had yet to be resolved. There was no widespread agreement on the duration of PA training programs; that is, the programs ranged from six weeks to five years. Inclusion of required years of prior training as prerequisites for many programs would extend the length of some programs up to a total of six years. There was no agreement on the preferred recruitment source. Some programs felt prior health- or medical-related experience and education were important in that their programs built upon this prior knowledge; other programs were more self-contained providing all the health experience and education required. Thus, ex-medical corpsmen, nurses, allied health professionals, high school graduates, college graduates, and the like were all seen as acceptable recruits by some of the programs. No general agreement existed on the appropriate role and functions to be fulfilled by the PA. The legal status of the PA had yet to be determined. Although acceptance of the initial PA graduates by physicians, other health professionals, and patients was promising, long range acceptance was still in question.

The research presented here addressed itself to many of the unresolved issues surrounding the introduction of the PA. Some special emphasis was placed on the issue of acceptability. Would the PA prove acceptable to the medical profession and thus be widely used in an effective and efficient manner? Would a PA be viewed as a competitor with, or a complement to, existing health professionals? Would the services of a PA be welcomed by consumers?

TIMELINESS OF THE RESEARCH

Although the birth of the PA concept took place in the early and mid-1960s it was not until the late 1960s and early 1970s that the PA received substantial attention on a national scale. Only after publication of the NAS report did the American Medical Association (AMA) in December 1970 adopt a working definition for the term "physician's assistant."[9] In fact, the AMA's ultimate endorsement of the nonnurse-PA concept came only after efforts to develop a nurse-PA were thwarted by professional nursing.

In December 1969, the AMA (after clearing its proposal with the American Hospital Association but not the American Nurses' Association) suggested that a means to expand health services would be to have nurses practice medicine under the supervision of a physician.[10] Subsequently, in February 1970, AMA Executive Vice-president Ernest B. Howard stated that a way of expanding physician's services would be to provide 100, 000 nurses with "modest additional training" (primarily through a kind of apprentice training given by their physician-employers) in order to prepare them to assume a PA role.[11] Howard's speech was followed a few days later by the endorsement of such a proposal by the AMA Board of Trustees. Deploring the AMA's unilateral action, the president of the American Nurses' Association (ANA), Dorothy Cornelius, asserted:

It is not the prerogative of one profession to speak for another. We strongly object to this unilateral action by the AMA, that they would attempt to meet the physician shortage by compounding the shortage of nurses.[12]

The National League for Nursing's (NLN) reaction to the AMA proposal was similar. Some of the significant aspects of the NLN's position included the following:

. . . the integrity of each health profession and its contribution to health care must be respected. . . . Any proposal for the expansion of the nurse's role should emanate from nursing, not from outside the profession. . . . It is not the role of a school of nursing to prepare a physician's assistant.[13]

Earlier that month (February 1970), the ANA had issued a statement on new health careerists calling for meetings between medicine and nursing ". . . to examine together their respective roles and those of each of the assistants utilized in medical and nursing care."[14] This statement was in keeping with a recommendation of a three-year study of nursing education and practice which had just been completed in January 1970, by the National Commission for the Study of Nursing and Nursing Education.[15] Noting the need for role articulation for all health practitioners, the commission's report (commonly known as the Lysaught Report) recommended the development of national and state joint practice commissions between medicine and nursing

to discuss and make recommendations concerning the congruent roles of the physician and the nurse in providing quality health care, with particular attention to the rise of the nurse master clinician; the introduction of the physician's assistant; the increased activity of other professions in areas long assumed to be the concern solely of the physician and/or the nurse.[16]

In March 1970, an official meeting was held between medical and nursing leaders; as a result of this meeting an ANA-NLN-AMA ad hoc committee to discuss the changing relationships between these two major health professions was instituted. The following year (August 1971), this committee began the difficult task of establishing the national and state joint practice commissions as recommended in the Lysaught Report.

In June 1970, the AMA Board of Trustees and House of Delegates approved a position statement on medicine and nursing in the 1970s.[17] Stating six objectives for the development of more optimal physician-nurse relationships, the role of the nurse as an "associate" of the physician was stressed. As such, the nurse, albeit under the overall supervision of the physician, would share a substantial amount of authority with him.[18] However, the AMA again reiterated its previous position with regard to the medical aspects of an expanded nurse role; after a short period of intensive training, nurses should ". . . assume greater medical service responsibility under the supervision of physicians."[19]

In referring to this official position paper, Charles L. Leedham, Chairman of the AMA Committee on Nursing, contended that "the concept of the nurse as the physician's assistant is as old as the relationship between nurses and physicians."[20] Leedham, however, was quick to assert that there was a difference between the nurse-PA and the nonnurse-PA; the nonnurse-PA was viewed as a complement to the nurse:

> The nonnurse physician's assistant is an individual trained for a specific task, a set of tasks, or a specific area of operation and responsibility. Such training is not intended to replace nursing functions.[21]

The ANA, however, was not in agreement with the AMA position. In October 1970, Eileen M. Jacobi, Executive Director of the ANA, explained:

> . . . physicians have the right to develop individuals who will assist them in the routine technical aspects of medical practice. However, we do not believe, as the AMA does, that this is an appropriate role for registered nurses, as this would be a waste of nurse manpower.[22]

Although not objecting to the expansion of the nurses' role, including an increased responsibility for many medical activities, the ANA did not want these new nurse practitioners (NPs) to be known as PAs. However, in the early years of the development of both of these new health professionals (nonnurse-PAs and NPs), both medical and nursing publications referred to both groups (in a generic sense) as PAs.[23]

Thus, in 1970, the issue of the PA was in the forefront of discussions between the two major health professions. In addition, national manpower policy advocated the introduction of the PA into the health field. The PA concept, which had developed so unobtrusively in the 1960s, became a focal point of controversy in the early 1970s.

NOTES

1. Rashi Fein, "An Economist's View: Medical Manpower—A Continuing Crisis," Journal of the American Medical Association 201, no. 6 (September 1967): 172.

2. V. R. Fuchs, "Can the Traditional Practice of Medicine Survive," Archives of Internal Medicine 125 (1970): 154-56.

3. Chris N. Theodore, "Physician Support Personnel in the 70's—Economic Implications," Journal of the American Medical Association 214, no. 7 (November 1970): 1302.

4. Harvey E. Estes, "The Critical Shortage—Physician and Supporting Personnel," Annals of Internal Medicine 69, no. 5 (November 1968): 959.

5. Ibid., pp. 957-62; Fein, op. cit., pp. 171-73; Malcolm C. Todd, "Medical Manpower and the Emergence of New Professions," Texas Medicine 68, no. 10 (October 1972): 60-64.

6. Fein, op. cit., p. 173.

7. National Academy of Sciences, New Members of the Physician's Health Team: Physician's Assistants (Washington, D. C.: The Academy, 1970), pp. 1-14.

8. Paraphrase, ibid., pp. 3-4.

9. Todd, op. cit., p. 60.

10. National Commission for the Study of Nursing and Nursing Education, An Abstract for Action (New York: McGraw-Hill, 1970), p. 88.

11. "AMA Unveils Surprise Plan to Convert R. N. into Medic," American Journal of Nursing 70, no. 4 (April 1970): 691.

12. Ibid.

13. Margaret E. Walsh, "Officially Speaking. . .," RN 33, no. 10 (October 1970): 86, 88.

14. Eileen M. Jacobi, "Officially Speaking. . .," RN 33, no. 10 (October 1970): 57.

15. National Commission for the Study of Nursing and Nursing Education, op. cit., pp. 1-167.

16. Ibid., p. 89.

17. American Medical Association's Committee on Nursing, "Medicine and Nursing in the 1970's: A Position Statement," Journal of the American Medical Association 213, no. 11 (September 1970): 1881-1883.

18. Ibid., p. 1883.

19. Ibid., p. 1881.

20. Charles L. Leedham, "Officially Speaking. . .," RN 33, no. 10 (October 1970): 90.

21. Ibid.

22. Jacobi, op. cit., p. 82.

23. "The Physician's Assistant Programs," RN 33, no. 10 (October 1970): 43-46; Joseph Kadish and James W. Long, "The Training of Physician Assistants: Status and Issues," Journal of the American Medical Association 212, no. 6 (May 1970): 1049.

CHAPTER

2

THE RESEARCH METHODOLOGY

STUDY DESIGN

The study design was an exploratory one with some descriptive elements. An exploratory study, as defined in the present context, is an attempt ". . . to gain familiarity with a phenomenon and to achieve new insights into it, in order to formulate a more precise research problem and to develop appropriate testable hypotheses."[1] Specifically, the author's study was exploratory in that it investigated a relatively unknown phenomenon; that is, it examined a new, and in many respects an untested, health professional—the physician's assistant.

Some elements of the study were descriptive in that an attempt was made to ". . . estimate the proportion of people in a specified population who hold certain views or attitudes. . ." toward a particular phenomenon.[2] The research was designed to identify the attitudes of two study populations toward the PA with reference to many of the pertinent issues surrounding his introduction into the health system.

There are three methods usually employed in conducting exploratory studies.[3] First, a review of the literature is valuable; this review increases the researcher's awareness of the problem and suggests tentative research questions. As is customary in an exploratory study, no formal hypotheses were tested in the author's study; rather, based upon an initial review of the relevant PA literature and upon lines of inquiry suggested by the theoretical framework discussed in Chapter 3, a series of research questions were formulated. The questions were a means of specifying relationships which might prove to be areas for further investigation. For example, based on the relationship between crisis perception and willingness to accept an innovation as noted in the diffusion of innovation literature, if the respondent perceived that a crisis situation existed with regard to a shortage of health manpower, would he more often have a positive attitude toward the use of a PA than a respondent who did not perceive the situation to be of crisis proportions? Based on the sociology of occupation literature, what are the characteristics of a nurse who viewed the PA as a complement to her own role on the health team as opposed to seeing the new position as a threat to her own career development? Finally, based on health manpower literature, to what extent will the physicians perceive their functions to be transferable ones?

The research questions were then used to guide the construction of the survey instruments used in both the author's national and local studies. Finally, the results of the study were used in the development of "working hypotheses" to provide the basis for more extensive research.

The second method employed in an exploratory study is to survey people who have had practical experience with the problem being investigated. In order to comply with this requirement, the first study population was identified; that is, a list was compiled of all operative and planned PA programs which the author was able to identify as of September 1970. A short open-end questionnaire was constructed, pretested, modified on the basis of the pretest, and mailed to 33 operative and 10 planned PA programs in late 1970 (see Appendix A). In July 1973, a second questionnaire was constructed and sent to the original programs in the 1970 sample (see Appendix B). Therefore, at two different time periods using two different instruments, the attitudes of those most familiar with the PA concept were examined.

The analysis of a local indepth case study is a third method employed in exploratory research.

> Scientists working in relatively unformulated areas, where there is little experience to serve as a guide, have found the intensive study of selected examples to be a particularly fruitful method for stimulating insights and suggesting hypotheses for research.[4]

It was for this reason that part of the author's investigation of the PA concept involved an examination of the potential acceptability of <u>one type</u> of PA. Specifically, a second study population was chosen composed of all providers of obstetrical services in a medium-sized southern city (12 physicians, 37 hospital obstetrical nurses, and 11 office obstetrical nurses) and a selected purposive sample of patients (expectant mothers). A separate questionnaire was constructed for each of the samples in this second study population. Utilizing

Utilizing the case study approach, the researcher must have an attitude of seeking rather than testing.[5] A suggested means of putting this approach into operation is to select ". . . individuals who represent different positions in the social structure. . . to produce a different view of the situation they are reflecting."[6] Thus, the second study population included obstetricians, obstetrical nurses, and obstetrical patients; these categories represent the potential employer, the coworker, and the recipient of the obstetrical PA's care, respectively.

DATA COLLECTION

Five questionnaires were constructed for use in the data collection phase of the survey. All were pretested and, as a result of each pretest, modified. The first national survey questionnaire was composed of 11 open-end questions sent in the form of a letter to each of the operative and planned PA programs in the sample (see Appendix A). The second questionnaire, used in the 1973 restudy of PA programs, was a structured variation of the 1970 questionnaire (see Appendix B). The other three instruments were used in the local case study of the obstetrical PA (see Appendixes C-E). The physicians' and nurses' questionnaires contained many similar questions in order that many responses of these two groups could be compared in the subsequent analysis. The patients' questionnaire, although containing references to many of the same substantive issues, was a significantly shortened and simplified version of the former two.

Both national questionnaires were mailed; several follow-up letters and postcards were sent to those who did not respond after an appropriate period. The local physician questionnaires were distributed by one of the obstetricians who volunteered to help the researcher with her study. The nurses' questionnaires were individually delivered and explained by the researcher. The nurses then returned the completed questionnaire by mail. Telephone calls were used to follow up those physicians and nurses who did not respond within a reasonable length of time. The patient questionnaires were given to the patients in four separate sessions of a community prenatal class. Identical explanations were given to each class prior to distributing the questionnaires in order to explain the study and the concept of a PA. The patients were given an opportunity to ask questions regarding PAs. The patients returned the completed questionnaires at the end of the class.

RESPONSE RATE

National Surveys

Of the 33 operative PA programs in the 1970 survey, there were only five nonrespondents. Of the 28 respondents, two did not supply sufficient information for inclusion in the study; thus there was a 79 percent usable response rate of the operative PA programs in 1970.

Of the 10 planned programs, only one did not respond. Three responded that, since they had received no funding, plans for their programs had been temporarily suspended; one other program responded but the information was insufficient to include in the analysis. Therefore, although the initial response rate was 90 percent, the usable response rate was 50 percent for the planned programs. The total usable response rate for both operative and planned PA programs in 1970 was 72 percent (see Appendix F).

In the 1973 restudy, using a total sample size of 43 programs, the initial response rate was 63 percent (27 programs) including a 64 percent response (nine programs) from the NP (nurse practitioner) portion of the sample and a 62 percent response (18 programs) from the PA portion of the sample. However, one 1970 operative NP program had been discontinued, plans for one PA program had been dropped, and one PA program response was incomplete; therefore, the total usable response rate in 1973 was 56 percent (see Appendix F).

In the author's 1970 national survey, the program respondents consisted of 26 operative and five planned PA programs.* The respondent group in the 1973 resurvey was composed of 16 PA programs and eight NP programs. In 1973, some of these early PA and NP programs had already been functioning for a period of eight years, although most programs had been operative for five years or less. The majority of the early programs (both PA and NP) had an educational base in a medical school or medical center. The length of study most frequently required in PA programs in 1973 was 24 months, although two of the programs required four academic years to complete. NP program length varied from four months to 18 months since all required a nursing education as a prerequisite. As of late 1973, 14 of the 16 PA program respondents reported 634 current students (170 of which were in different phases of one four-year program) and 369 graduates (five of the more recent programs had no graduates) of which 352 were currently employed in PA positions; thus, 95 percent of the reported graduates of nine of the earliest PA programs were actively engaged in their new career. The eight NP programs in the 1973 study reported 196 current students and 713 graduates of which 635 were actively functioning in NP roles; thus, 89 percent of the graduates of eight early NP programs were active practitioners functioning in an expanded health provider role.

---

*As explained in Chapter 4, the 1970 study adopted a broad generic interpretation of the term PA; consequently, several NR programs were classified as PA programs. Using more current terminology (1973), the 1970 "PA" respondent group was comprised of 20 PA programs and 11 NP programs. In the 1973 resurvey, the unique qualities of each of these new health professionals is acknowledged and the data for each are separately analyzed.

As one would anticipate, the vast majority of NP students and graduates in the programs were female while the vast majority of PA students and graduates were male. However, there were significant variations among the PA programs in the male-female ratio with three programs having a ratio equal to or greater than 20 to 1 and five having a ratio equal to or less than 3 to 2. The ratio of Black, Indian, Chicano to white in the NP student and graduate population varied from a low of 0 to 1 to a high of 3 to 2 while a similar ratio in PA programs varied from a low of 0 to 1 to a high of 6 to 1. On the average, NP students were somewhat older than PA students; the average age of a NP recruit was 33 years while the average age of a PA recruit was 26 years.

Local Case Study

The local case study population was composed of the three major referents of the obstetrical PA: obstetricians, obstetrical nurses, and obstetrical patients. The physician sample included the total population of physicians who offered obstetrical services in the selected community; as such, it included 10 specialists in obstetrics and gynecology and two general practitioners. Of the 10 specialists, seven were actively engaged in obstetrical practice and three had within the past year limited their practices to gynecology. Of the 12 possible physician respondents, eight responded, giving a total usable response rate of 67 percent.

The nurse component of the local study included the total population of obstetrical nurses—both RNs (registered nurses) and LPNs (licensed practical nurses)—in the community. This included nurses who worked in obstetricians' offices and in the obstetrical services of the two local general hospitals. The entire population included 37 hospital nurses and 11 office nurses. Of the 37 hospital nurses, 32 responded: a response rate of 86 percent. Of the 11 office nurses, eight responded: a response rate of 73 percent. The total usable response rate for the obstetrical nurses (both hospital and office) was 83 percent.

The third element of the local study population consisted of expectant mothers who attended community parenthood classes. This last group of respondents did not meet the criteria of random sampling; it involved nonprobability sampling since it included only a particular subgroup of the potential patient population: the expectant mothers who attended several selected sessions of the parenthood classes. It should be acknowledged that there is a certain selectivity in the expectant mothers who choose to attend such classes as opposed to those mothers who choose not to attend. The classes were composed of four formal sessions plus a tour of the relevant facilities of the local hospitals. The first two classes of the series were concerned with the early prenatal period; therefore, the patients who attended these sessions were generally early in their pregnancies. The second two classes covered essential aspects of childbirth, labor and delivery, and infant care; thus, the patients who attended these classes were generally in the more advanced stages of their pregnancies.

Questionnaires were administered during four sessions of the classes; two were during the second class, one during the fourth class and one was given to a session of the classes specially scheduled during a local general hospital's antenatal clinic hours and designed to attract predominately clinic patients. By selecting sessions during different phases of the course and by including a clinic session, it was hoped that the patient respondent group would constitute a diverse sample which might be fairly representative of obstetrical patients in the community. The total number of usable responses was 45 out of a possible sample size of 47, resulting in a 96 percent response rate.

Although the number of respondents in the local case study was comparatively small, the sample's unique aspects made it particularly valuable for the total research effort. One such unique asset of the local sample was that it included all relevant subgroups of the health care community that the proposed type of PA being investigated would serve. In this way, the total potential acceptability of the obstetrical PA could be examined. In addition, one must remain cognizant of the aims of exploratory research. The total study (including both national and local surveys) was an effort to interrelate selected aspects of the literature, the practical experience obtained by the programs involved in the development of a new type of health manpower, and an intensive examination of the potential acceptability of one type of PA in a medium-sized southern city. In sum, the study utilized the major methods of exploratory research; thus, its ultimate value should be its usefulness in providing some working hypotheses and a firm basis for future more extensive research in the area.

NOTES

1. Claire Sellitz et al., Research Methods in Social Relations, 2nd ed. (New York: Henry Holt, 1960), p. 50.
2. Ibid., p. 65.
3. Ibid., pp. 53-64.
4. Ibid., p. 59.
5. Ibid., p. 60.
6. Ibid., p. 63.

CHAPTER

3

A DISCUSSION OF THEORETICALLY RELEVANT LITERATURE: INNOVATIONS AND RESISTANCE TO CHANGE, ORGANIZATIONS AND CONFLICT, AND HEALTH MANPOWER

INTRODUCTION

As introduced above, the research presented in this study (Chapters 4-6) is exploratory and descriptive. As such, it does not rely upon a well-formulated and highly integrated theory; there are exceedingly few theories of this nature in the social sciences and health fields. In fact, these areas are often viewed as being pervaded by atheoretical materials. The question of acceptability of new health professionals, such as the PA, is one that is affected by a great many variables and is relevant to numerous publics. However, related research need not be atheoretical. In addition to her own observations made as a health worker and researcher, the author was guided by, and hopefully contributes to, several established theoretical frameworks.

Existing research concerning the PA can be theoretically characterized as fragmented. Such fragments (or empirical generalizations, if you prefer) will only become of genuine value when they are drawn together. The author believes that the theoretical avenues discussed herein are central to a better understanding of health care delivery and, specifically, to the PA within this system; she also hopes that this exploratory research will contribute to the synthesis necessary to provide a suitable theoretical grounding for future contributions to the study of health care provision. Of particular importance to the organization, analysis, and discussion of the research presented is the social science literature concerning: (1) the diffusion of innovations and those general obstacles to implementing change; (2) change and conflict within organizations; and (3) health manpower research. These areas are selectively and briefly discussed below—keeping in mind that many volumes have been written on each subject.

DIFFUSION OF INNOVATIONS

There is a large body of behavioral science literature devoted to the diffusion and adoption of innovations.* Within these studies an innovation is viewed as

> . . . an idea, practice, or object perceived as new by an individual. . . [or group]. . . . "New" in an innovative idea need not be simply new knowledge. . . . The "newness" aspect of an innovation may be expressed in knowledge, in attitude, or regarding a decision to use it.[1]

The response of health professionals and patients to the PA is certainly an issue which is concerned with an innovation in the health field, particularly as it pertains to the third type of "newness" above. Whereas the idea of an assistant to physicians (other than the nurse and existing allied health professionals) is not objectively new, the actual incorporation of such an innovative role into the system of health care delivery via special training programs established specifically for the PA is new. At the time the case study reported in Chapter 6 was conducted, no obstetrician in the study community was employing a PA. Clearly the concept and use of an obstetrical PA (with which the local study dealt) could be considered an innovation in the study community.

Although much of innovations research has been conducted on the adoption or rejection of agricultural or educational ideas and practices (particularly the former), there is an established research tradition within medical sociology that has dealt with this issue. Probably the classic study in the latter field was conducted by Katz, Menzel, and Coleman at the Columbia University Bureau of Applied Social Research.[2] Among other findings, the researchers discovered that physicians who were early adopters of newly developed antibiotics were more likely to be characterized by a cosmopolite orientation and to be opinion leaders in their profession than were noninnovators. In the twenty years since the "Columbia Drug Study," there has been a significant amount of further research in the innovation area; many findings have been substantiated over a variety of settings. Some of those that appear most relevant to the adoption of the PA within the health care system are mentioned below.

---

*Perhaps the best single source book for studies concerning the adoption of innovation is: Everett M. Rogers and F. Floyd Shoemaker, Communication of Innovations: A Cross-Cultural Approach (New York: Free Press, 1971). The following discussion relies upon this reference rather extensively.

One factor that obviously plays an important role in the adoption of innovations is the degree to which a given innovation is perceived as being better than the idea (arrangement, device, or the like) it is to supersede. One factor that has been found to emphasize the relative advantage of the new over the old is the existence of a crisis. Although not universally true, most agricultural research has shown that the presence of a crisis accelerates the adoption of new practices.[3]

The compatibility a proposed innovation has with current practice and tradition is highly relevant to whether or not it is adopted and, if adopted, to the rate at which it is adopted. There are at least three respects in which an innovation may or may not be compatible: it may or may not be compatible with previously introduced ideas, with client needs for innovation, and with sociocultural values and beliefs.[4] With regard to the first two considerations, studies suggest that more compatible innovations pave the way for future less compatible changes, and "when felt needs are met, a faster rate of adoption should occur."[5]

A proposed change that is not compatible with well-entrenched and pervasive values stands a poor chance of being adopted or, at least, its rate of adoption is unlikely to be rapid. Most studies that dramatically demonstrate this are those conducted by anthropologists in so-called underdeveloped areas as well as those research projects examining the efforts of agricultural extension workers. Although some may question the relevance of this literature to a study of the receptivity of new health workers, there are some interesting parallels to be noted. The one-to-one doctor-patient relationships has become, for a very large portion of the U. S. population, a cultural expectation. A proposal which might appear to substitute another health worker for the physician is one which is incompatible with this expectation. A good deal of research indicates that those who adapt most readily to change are more likely to belong to or identify with groups and positions which have been described as being primarily modern rather than traditional in orientation.[6]

There is still another attribute that proposed innovations may possess which can prove especially significant to further research on the PA concept. This aspect has been given the somewhat awkward label of "trialability." "Trialability is the degree to which an innovation may be experimented with on a limited basis."[7] In essence, if you can adopt an innovation a little at a time (in installments, if you will) it will be adopted more quickly than innovations which are not as "divisible." The perception of trialability has been found to be particularly important in the decisions of the early adopters. This concept will be readily recognized as closely related to the above concept of compatibility; for example, if an idea can be shown to be both compatible and divisible, it has a particularly high potential of being adopted. Perhaps, on a national scope, we are now witnessing the gradual adoption of the PA via a trial basis; that is, the PA is being allowed entry into the health field, but his activities are still very circumscribed in many practice settings (for example, the hospital).

There are many variables which have been found to closely correlate with the early adoption of innovations. Recently, these have been categorized in accord with whether or not they are primarily socioeconomic or communicative in nature.[8] (Everett Rogers and Floyd Shoemaker also discuss personality variables and their relationship to early adoption; this is a legitimate area of analysis, but it is one the author elected not to examine or discuss.) Among the socioeconomic variables which would appear to be of likely significance to studies of new health professionals, findings show that earlier adopters are of higher social status than their counterparts and that they are upwardly striving within their own occupation (profession). Additionally, early adopters have larger scale operations, tend to be oriented toward increasing economic profits (as opposed to operating a "subsistence" venture), and are more likely to specialize within their given occupation.

One of the most important contingencies to consider when explaining who will and who will not favor a given innovation is the communication behavior of the persons involved. Obviously one must be aware of a proposed change before he can have the option of adopting. Beyond this, there are several other communication variables associated with a favorable disposition to innovation—a cosmopolite character has already been mentioned above. Early adopters have greater contact with those who propose the change in question (change agents), and they are more frequently involved in interpersonal (face-to-face) communications with other members of their field than nonadopters. Those oriented to adoption generally seek and acquire more information concerning innovations and thereby have greater knowledge of the latest ideas, implements, and so on than do their nonadopter counterparts.

Herbert Lionberger, in his book Adoption of New Ideas and Practices, provides several other generalizations which may prove relevant to the adoption of the PA. Local leadership, for example, is expected to uphold and to adhere to locally accepted standards; if these standards call for a cautious approach to the adoption of new ideas, the local leaders will not likely become early advocates of adoption.[9] It has also been shown that identity with or membership in a formal group may affect an individual's attitude toward an innovation if the group has taken a position on the issue; however "to the extent that norms conducive to rational inquiry and change. . . are accepted as group norms and are internalized individually, the group's influence on members will likely be conducive to change."[10]

Finally, whereas much of the research indicates that there is a strong correlation between formal education and early adoption, it has also been suggested that ". . . education may merely create a supposedly favorable mental atmosphere for the acceptance of new practices."[11] In other words, even though education has been found to be an important factor in promotion of adoption, knowledge of individuals' education is not sufficient to predict early adoption; in some cases, a considerable amount of education may not prove necessary for one to become an innovator.

The preceding selective discussion of variables that have been noted to be positively related to adoption of innovations is hardly all inclusive; there are other factors which could be discussed (and many yet to be discovered) that should lend to a fuller explanation of the willingness to innovate. As perceived within the context of the social science research on innovations, the receptivity (or lack of it) shown the concept and actual employment of the PA presents a heretofore unexamined issue. Looking to the immediate future, the rich literature on innovations in fields of other substantive interests may provide the initial theoretical foundation for research investigating this new health professional. Numerous working hypotheses could be generated regarding the acceptance of the PA by the medical profession drawing upon the private physician's homologue in the vast agricultural innovations literature—the commercial farmer. For example, referring back to the discussion of socioeconomic characteristics of early adopters, one might hypothesize that private physicians who are among the first to employ PAs would probably be specialists who are upwardly striving within their profession and currently have a comparatively large lucrative practice, which they were actively attempting to expand.

If research on the PA is incorporated into an innovations framework, it should also prove a challenge for this tradition. Whereas much research on innovation has dealt with the adoption of a new idea or practice by one party, the successful acceptance of the PA clearly necessitates receptivity of the new professional role not only by physician-employers and institutions, but also by members of the other health professions, such as nurses, as well as by the patient group. Although it is well documented that the adoption of a new technology often has far-reaching and unanticipated consequences for the sociocultural system, the proposed widespread integration of PAs into the current health care system obviates any doubts that the change in question will have an impact upon the basic organization of health care delivery, thus touching on social, cultural, and psychological aspects of all groups concerned.

THREE OBSTACLES TO CHANGE

Much of the above may be viewed as primarily relevant to the physicians, hospitals, clinics, and other groups which will consider the adoption of PAs as members of their health delivery teams. In the next section, there is provided discussion of some of the general organizational (professional) factors which may facilitate or impede acceptance of the PA. However, as suggested above, the potential clients (patients) of this new health care worker will also play a role in his acceptance. Several years ago, the prominent anthropologist,

George Foster, outlined the major barriers which inhibit members of the community from accepting proposed innovations.* These barriers are viewed both from the perspective of the people considering change and as major problems for the agents who advocate adoption. The three are characterized as being primarily cultural, social, and psychological.

Cultural Barriers

What are the major cultural barriers to be considered? Reliance upon tradition and an avoidance of the novel is one. For example, outreach prenatal classes and clinics have often failed in rural America partially because tradition suggests that a pregnancy is an intimate issue to be kept within the family and that older women (particularly the expectant woman's mother or mother-in-law) are the appropriate recognized advisors on matters relating to childbirth. Might not the traditional felt and expected doctor-patient intimacy that has become established in mainstream America thwart ready acceptance of a nonphysician performing many of the tasks fulfilled previously only by doctors? If certain members of the community feel their pride has been offended by a given change or the way in which it is offered them, one can certainly expect a negative response. Governmental programs that have sought to give advice or give or sell inexpensively food stuffs have frequently failed to anticipate the negative (nonreceptive) consequences. If health services provided by the PA were to have the misfortune to be perceived as second-class care, one could predict a similar lack of acceptance. Ethnocentrism, with its strong status quo orientation, is a cultural universal that makes all people resistant and suspect of change, especially when proposed change is viewed as emanating from an "out group" idea or practice. The PA, as a

---

*Many of the major concepts from that outline are utilized in the following paragraphs. See George M. Foster, Traditional Cultures and the Impact of Technological Change (New York: Harper, 1962). As indicated by the title, Foster's major focus is upon the impediments to western technological change found among people of the modernizing world. However, the three general barriers he discusses are also relevant to the adoption of proposed changes in any community. This may well be particularly true for families from rural areas and low income urban neighborhoods; as discussed in Chapter 5, these are two areas that a number of current PA training programs emphasize as primary service populations. However, it is unlikely that these factors would only prove applicable in such settings.

nonphysician practicing health care with varying degrees of independent judgment, has little precedent in the United States; consequently, early attempts to promote the PA concept often referred to such independent practitioners as the feldsher in the USSR and the assistant medical officer in Africa. Such analysis could very well prove counter productive due to the considerable likelihood of arousing ethnocentric reactions not only from potential patient groups, but also from existing health care providers.

Social Barriers

Closely linked with the values and belief systems of a community are the ways in which groups are interrelated. This structure may also facilitate certain social barriers to the adoption of change. Although kinship relationships are fairly well recognized as highly important in developing areas, their influence is sometimes overlooked in modern urbanized society. Whereas decisions regarding health care are often viewed as individual-rational ones (an individual seeks medical care when he feels ill), actually such decisions might more appropriately be viewed as being made for an individual in conjunction with one or more family members. Identification of an illness, preliminary diagnosis, whom to consult, and so on, are rarely unilateral decisions; they are validated by the family as a group. The successful promotion of the PA will partially depend upon the extent to which this new practitioner appeals to the family as a unit.

Factionalism of some proportion is another fact of life in any community or neighborhood. Community bifurcation along extended kin lines ("feudin'") has won itself a romantic role in American folklore, but factionalism for the proponent of innovation can present itself as a very real, if less dramatic, challenge. Such splits may occur on the basis of such characteristics as class, ethnicity, age, or politics; invariably adoption of the innovation or sponsorship of the agent of change by one group is met with suspicion and initial resistance by the other. On a number of substantive issues pertaining to proposed innovation, the community and change agents alike are faced with the fact that there exists no formal decision-making structure—no person or persons capable or willing to speak for the locality on the proposal in question. Ad hoc committees sometimes arise under these conditions, but frequently advocates must literally convince every concerned or potentially concerned resident in a sizeable portion of the community. Proponents of major changes in health care delivery should be aware of these structural realities.

Psychological Barriers

Foster labels his third category of barriers to change psychological.* A first variable of concern is the way in which the innovation and especially its promoters are perceived. If this perception is characterized by feelings such as mistrust, suspicion, or hostility, it will scarcely lead to facile adoption. In an era characterized by ever-increasing bureaucratization, a spiraling cost of living, costly medical insurance affording insufficient benefits, and so on, many people are simply suspect of any proposal that promises to provide them with greater health and welfare benefits. With the public's confidence in public and private spokesmen and institutions somewhat undermined, its receptivity toward a new health practitioner, sponsored in part by these parties, is unpredictable. A second barrier also depends heavily on the advocates of change; the nature of communication between change agents and potential adopters is widely recognized as an area in which many costly mistakes have been committed. If medical and health institutions are to actively promote and employ the PA, then patient receptivity would be improved by better professional-client communication. Conversely, failure to adequately explain the role that the PA is to play would substantially reduce his chances for acceptance.

The cultural, social, and psychological variables discussed above were couched in terms of factors impeding the acceptance of proposed innovations; it should be kept in mind that a lack of these conditions should thereby enhance receptivity. The next section briefly outlines the major components of social organization and discusses sources of intergroup and intragroup conflict—both of considerable relevance to a better understanding of tensions and change within the health care systems.

SOCIAL ORGANIZATION AND CONFLICT

Components of Social Organization

Understanding the principal components of social organization—the major concern of the discipline of sociology—and its relationship to organizational conflict is a level of analysis well suited to students

---

*These factors do not involve personality dynamics and might be as easily thought of as both socio-psychological and communication variables.

interested in explaining interaction within the health care system. In the abstract, social organization may be said to comprise four chief components: norms, roles, sanctions, and social ranking.* Norms are simply the rules which govern human interactions. Many norms have specialized application; that is, they are relevant to certain categories of members in a given system (for example, doctors, nurses, technicians). Obviously, in order to be effective, norms must be supported by the consensus of the members of the organization. There is a very basic paradox involving norms: they at once both reduce personal freedom and make personal interactions less complicated and confusing.

Roles designate the rights, duties, and obligations of group members. In formal systems such as a hospital, the official roles are often explicitly stated. Role allocation lies at the very basis of division of labor; there are, for example, specialized expectations for the different groups of health providers within the system. The behaviors and anticipations of these workers are organized by mutual understanding of the place each has in the health care system of roles. Leadership within any system may be viewed as arising in order to coordinate various roles so that the system's major goals are best fulfilled. Health care is not found within a single system in the United States; it comprises many different professions, agencies, corporations, and branches of government. One might suggest that, to the extent that there exists a leadership crisis in the health field, it is due to the fact there is no intergroup leadership with recognized authority to coordinate roles between groups.

Positive and negative sanctions (social control) are the primary means by which stability is maintained in human groups. (This is frequently interpreted as being an orientation toward the status quo, but stability may also be maintained within a system undergoing change—a major challenge to leadership.) Sanctions are applied in order to make certain that system members: (1) abide by group norms; (2) perform their respective roles adequately; and (3) coordinate activities to maximize the achievement of group goals. Regardless of the manipulative implications for the use of sanctions to regulate human interaction, its use is well recognized within formal organizations; the heads of such groups are respected (as well as feared) because they are vested with the authority to administer punishment and reward.

Social ranking (stratification) refers to the phenomenon within social organizations whereby various roles (once institutionalized) become ranked hierarchically according to their degree of status.

---

*While a majority of sociologists would generally agree that these components constitute the basic concepts of social organization, this particular discussion very closely follows the excellent presentation in Melvin L. DeFleur, William V. D'Antonio, and Lois B. DeFleur, Sociology: Man in Society (Glenview, Illinois: Scott Foresman, 1971).

Persons usually occupy high status positions for one of three reasons: (1) they are vested with greater authority than the majority; (2) their presumed talent is viewed as comparatively scarce; and (3) they have undergone a long period of demanding training. The latter two criteria are frequently mentioned as reasons for U. S. physicians receiving relatively high status and monetary reward. These criteria are not only employed for judging the relative position of roles, but are also used for selecting persons to fill these roles. Functionally oriented social scientists have frequently taken the position that ranking within a social system or society in general is ultimately integrative rather than divisive; that is, unequal distribution of status (wealth, power) is necessary to motivate individuals to fill certain roles and perform adequately. This view does not go unchallenged, but whatever position one takes in this regard, social ranking is at the heart of a good deal of system tension and conflict.

Types of Organizational Conflict

There are two types of organizational conflict, intergroup and intragroup, both of which are of obvious relevance to a health care system considering the adoption of a new health professional. This conflict may be categorized as stemming from various sources. There may exist, as there often does within institutions such as large businesses, universities, and hospitals, conflicting policies which require conflicting goals. For example, the team approach, often espoused as an appropriate relationship among health professionals within an institutional setting, implies goals not in keeping with the traditional hierarchy, which finds other workers subordinated to physicians. In actuality, integration of goals often means that the goals of one group (profession) do not completely negate the other. Very closely associated with conflicting goals, one often finds ineffective communication (or a complete breakdown of communication) leading to group tension and conflict. A group or network of groups must have and continue to have common goals, or else effective communication will break down or never be established. When the instrumental manifest goals of various health professions actually become secondary to the latent goal of self-aggrandizement, a lack of communication is likely to ensue.

Normative confusion is a very prevalent source of conflict, and this condition is most likely to occur during a crisis or at the point when a new order is impending. One finds a divergence of opinion within groups and between groups where spokesmen either behave in accord with current norms or choose to write anew or ignore behavioral guidelines. Certainly the various proposals regarding the PA indicate that there exists no unified perspective or integrated program that would govern the appropriate responsibilities of this new health provider and his relationship to other established professionals. If you add to this the confusion on the part of the prospective clients themselves, the result is that relatively few clearly know what to expect of the others.

Role conflict lies at the root of a good deal of intergroup and intragroup conflict. This tension develops within individuals in two ways: internal role conflict and external role conflict. The former pertains to the strains which are inherent in the role itself. Professional nurses, for example, may be seen as drawn between the presumed central role of direct (bedside) patient care, so emphasized in their philosophy of nursing orientation, and the ever increasing administrative tasks, which are required and which tend to be associated with greater status and reward. External role conflict is caused by the incompatible demands that are made by two or more roles. For example, health professionals, such as doctors and nurses, who become involved with the introduction of the PA into the health system may well find themselves divided on an allegiance to their own perceived professional self-interests and a commitment to a new coworker in health care delivery.

Disturbances in social ranking occur when the position and authority of one group is not recognized or is ranked differently by another. The college professor, for example, who encourages interpersonal peerlike relations with his students may be thought very popular with students, but this reduction in social distance can create ill feeling among his fellow professionals and make more difficult the role of scholar. With the introduction of the PA into the health system there arises the real possibility of a disturbance in the status hierarchy of a slightly different variety. What will be the relative ranking of the PA among other nonphysician health providers—particularly vis-a-vis professional nurses? The likelihood that many of these professionals will agree on such a ranking is questionable, as is any utopian assumption that they will ultimately be perceived and perceive each other as status equals.

Positive Functions of Conflict

Although conflict is usually responded to negatively, avoided by many, and admittedly generally unpleasant, its consequences should not be viewed as totally dysfunctional. Some of the conflict which has arisen and which will most certainly continue regarding the proper role of the PA could generate positive consequences. One of the positive functions conflict may perform is that of focusing attention upon a crucial issue and thus making widespread indifference less likely. Consequently influential third parties become more likely to take an active role in the resolution of issues when conflict surfaces. A second function of conflict is that which it often performs for a given group such as an occupation, a profession, or a team—the nurturing of group integration and cohesiveness. The presence of an external target that is perceived as threatening, frequently reduces intragroup disagreements and tensions and leads to more effective organization and performance.

A third positive function of conflict is perhaps the most obvious (or should be so): conflict is a major stimulus for change. As we move into the last quarter of the current century, we will have to contend with change ever increasingly exponential in character. This is markedly apparent when technology and cybernetics are considered. The social organization of society (including that of health care provision), however, must also attempt to keep pace. This implies that conflicts within these contexts will continue and probably increasingly be a way of life for the future.

The social sciences have recently, although at times grudgingly, recognized these positive functions of conflict. Lewis Coser was among the first "rediscoverers" of social conflict to cite the way in which it may stimulate responsive change in human organization:

> Conflict within and between groups in a society can prevent accommodations and habitual relations from progressively impoverishing creativity. The clash of values and interests, tensions between what is and what some groups feel ought to be. . . have been productive of vitality.[12]

Vital, effective social organizations must recognize the necessity of distinguishing between stability and stagnation. This has more recently been stated with a clear applicability to the U. S. system of health delivery:

> Stable groups change over time, just as stable individuals do. Indeed, unyielding resistance to change can sometimes boomerang and lead ultimately to a group's disintegration, for groups must adapt to changing circumstances if they are to be effective.[13]

Occupations

In addition to the literature on innovations and change, another subfield of sociology which should be especially relevant to future research on health professions is that of the sociology of occupations.*

---

*There are quite a number of good references in this area; two recent contributions are Ronald M. Pavalko, The Sociology of Occupations and Professions (Itasca, Illinois: Peacock, 1971) and Elliott A. Krause, The Sociology of Occupations (Boston: Little Brown, 1971). The

Most of the analyses found in this area employ one or both of the perspectives previously discussed: social organization or the causes and functions of conflict theory. This literature is not discussed at length in the present chapter. There are, however, several points which are well made by Elliott Krause and which seem appropriate to the substantive research topic—the PA as a new health professional.

Krause deemphasizes a "structure-function" approach and prefers to view occupations and professions from a processual perspective. In doing so, the focus is cast upon those factors that cause change, particularly as seen from positions of conflicts of interest. This, then, is obviously complementary to the perspective suggested above. Of course, it is far simpler to analyze the relationships between occupational groups (or between these groups and the citizenry) when they are well established. Emerging occupations present greater difficulties whether the strategy of analysis is predominantly that of functionalism or conflict. However, it is this very reason that will make research on the PA or similar emerging professions a major challenge to the sociology of occupations.

Another unique aspect of Krause's approach is that he does not fail to include the consumers of health care in his conflict of interest equation. Heretofore, most sociological analysis of the health industry and health professionals has emphasized conflicts among health providers themselves (nurses, general practitioners, specialists, technicians, hospital administrators, health insurance companies, and so on). An equally important (if not more important) issue ". . . is the conflict of interest between occupational groups in the health field and the public interest in the area of health. . . [or] the conflict between those who profit by the giving of health services and those who are the consumers of the services."[14] Whereas change and conflict are inevitable in the health care professions and the health field as a whole, this need not mean that the health care delivered to the public will necessarily be of better quality, more equitable across classes, more efficient, or less expensive. "It has become increasingly obvious to the citizen that the various conflict of interest battles which we have considered within the health field benefit him little, regardless of the outcome."[15] If, for example, the incorporation of a new health professional (such as the PA) does not ensure an increase in the general level of health care available, then all of the other considerations are at best academic. The health researcher, and particularly the planner, must not lose sight of this fact. While the American health industry continues to expand, the level of care for the "average" person continues to fall when the United States is compared to many European countries and

---

latter is of particular interest because it contains a separate chapter devoted to major issues of concern to professionals, workers, and the lay public in the area of health.

the Soviet Union. Major issues in the literature on health manpower are discussed in the next section.

HEALTH MANPOWER

Many spokesmen for various institutions in American society have noted with alarm the apparent shortage of health manpower when juxtaposed with the increased demand for health care. Some have gone as far as to suggest that we find ourselves in a crisis situation. Ironically, the health services industry is one of the largest in our nation, probably accounting for approximately 4 percent of the total civilian work force.* Growth within selected health occupations has been very rapid during the last decades, especially when compared to the overall population growth rate and the growth of the labor force as a whole. Between 1950 and 1960 the overall increase in employment for health professionals was 50.5 percent, relative to an 11.4 percent growth rate for the labor force and an 18.5 percent growth rate of the total population.[16]

The traditional health occupations of medicine, nursing, and dentistry, while accounting for a sizeable portion of the total employment within the health field, have recently experienced a relative decline. Whereas employment in these three health professions accounted for 49 percent of the total employment in the health field in 1950, in 1970 these professions represented only 37 percent of the total. Recent dramatic growth rates have particularly occurred in the fields of mental health manpower and in the so-called new health occupations such as occupational therapy and medical record technology.[17] Statements such as these emphasize the rates of growth and not absolute numbers; in terms of the latter, physicians, registered nurses, practical nurses, and aides, orderlies, and attendants still make up the sizeable majority of health workers.

When both numbers and relative growth rates of health manpower are considered, it may appear that supply is adjusting to demand. Perhaps then, the perceived manpower crisis is only a short-term one—an instance of a so-called transitory shortage. As such, the problem could be viewed as an unavoidable aspect of a system which was accommodating to change and, given sufficient lead time, would

---

*The job classification scheme used for the health services industry has been criticized for its analytical inefficiencies, which make difficult the measurement of the total numbers of those actually providing health services and changes in these numbers over time. For example, see Jeffrey H. Weiss, "A Job Classification Scheme for Health Manpower," Health Services Research 3, no. 1 (Spring, 1968): 48-64.

achieve an equilibrium wherein a sufficient supply of health workers would be educated to meet the demand for health care. Obviously the role of the PA and NP in this "marketplace model" can be alternatively interpreted in one of two ways. On the one hand, the use of these workers will diminish given the increased availability of physicians. On the other hand, the demand can equally well be seen as being met by these new workers who will be permanently incorporated into health services delivery. Whichever interpretation one favors, either is only comforting when you ignore the third and fourth aspects of the health manpower marketplace—distribution and utilization.

Distribution

The distribution of health manpower can be viewed from three perspectives: (1) locational or geographical distribution; (2) occupational distribution; and (3) specialty distribution within a given profession.[18] Some have asserted that our supply of health professionals is adequate to meet our health care needs. The 1959 Bane Committee Report[19] projected a total of 275, 000 physicians by 1965; the actual number of licensed physicians in 1965 was 305, 000. According to W. Lee Hansen, the apparent "surplus" of 30, 000 physicians was probably closer to only 6, 000, due to a faulty data system used for the 1959 baseline. Nonetheless, licensed physicians increased faster than had been projected, primarily due to the facts that more graduates were produced than anticipated, fewer physicians retired than assumed, and the influx of foreign physicians increased.[20] However, the mid-1960s was the very time when health delivery needs appeared particularly acute as suggested by the passage of legislation including Health Professions Education Assistance Act (1963), the Nurse Training Act (1964) and the Allied Health Professional Personnel Training Act (1966). The Health Professions Education Assistance Act provided approximately $100 million to increase the number of medical graduates over a three year period.

Geographic Distribution

One of the major reasons that such expenditures of effort and money did not begin to succeed in eradicating the physician shortage is the geographic maldistribution of physicians. For example, researchers have found that upper income areas have substantially larger numbers of physicians per capita than low income areas.[21] Why is this true? It is partially a product of the fact that upper income families can afford to visit physicians more often and have more expensive visits for which physicians are able to demand higher fees.

Eli Ginzberg and Harry I. Greenfield, in their respective books on health manpower, have questioned the desirability of increasing the numbers of such a highly paid commodity as the physician, precisely because of their maldistribution. Ginzberg reminds us that whenever there are scarce goods or services, people with more money will have greater access to them. He cites as one example the situation is Israel, a country with a high proportion of physicians per capita where clearly different groups of Israelites have differential access to good health care. In that country, there is more than one physician for every 500 persons; this compares with a ratio of one to every 814 persons in the United States. Nevertheless, rural coverage in Israel is inadequate even when some of the poorly served areas are less than two hours from a major city.[22]

Irene Butter noted that although the 1962 national ratio of physicians to the population (136 to 100, 000) was virtually identical to that of 1920 (134 to 100, 000), the range between the state having the lowest physician-to-population ratio and the state having the highest is greater than ever. This, then, clearly suggests an obviously increasing inequitable geographic distribution of physicians.[23] Professional nurses, in contrast, have experienced an increasing personnel-to-population ratio[24] and yet there continues to be problems of spatial maldistribution similar to that of physicians.[25] (Of course, a reasonably efficient optimum distribution of health professions need not necessarily suggest equal numbers of workers throughout the nation.)

Occupational Distribution

This refers to the mix of skills for the provision of health care. This mix changes through time, varies with practice settings, and exhibits regional variations. With respect to variations through time, in 1950, M. D. s together with osteopaths accounted for 13 percent of the total number of workers in 40 major health occupations. In 1970, these same workers represented eight percent of the total. Nurses accounted for 30 percent of the total employment in these 40 occupations in 1950, but only 25 percent in 1970. In contrast to the proportional representation of these two professions, in 1950 15 percent of employees in health occupations were aides, orderlies, and attendants; their proportion increased to 25 percent in 1970.[26] Such an altering of the mix in the health occupations may have implications for the way in which health care is provided. For example, could a partial explanation for this increase in the proportion of aides, orderlies, and attendants relative to physicians and nurses reflect a substitution of less costly lower skilled workers for the more costly higher skilled?

Practice settings also vary in their use of different types of health care personnel. The nursing profession provides an unusually vivid example of this. The vast majority of nurses in the United States are employed in hospitals rather than in a community setting (for example, in public health roles, in physicians' offices, schools, or industry). In fact, the ratio of hospital nurses to physicians is 35 times as great

(7.4 to 1) as the ratio of office-based nurses to physicians (.21 to 1).[27] In Great Britain, by way of contrast, the ratio of hospital nurses to physicians is 3 to 1, while office-based nurses to physicians is 1 to 1. Nurses in this latter instance are not employed by the physician; they are employed by the local health authority and assigned to a physician's office.[28] Presumably this should contribute to greater communication between physicians and nurses in Great Britain than in the United States.

There are two relevant questions pertaining to regional variations. One question regards the distribution of health occupations or the availability of health manpower. A second asks to what extent regions differ with respect to the delegation of health care tasks to nonphysicians. With respect to the former, it is clear the numbers of available professionals vary considerably by region. A good illustration of this is provided by a recent extensive survey of member pediatricians in the American Academy of Pediatrics (AAP) which highlighted some rather striking variations in the provision of ambulatory care available by region to infants and children. The data show that the southern states, when compared with New York City, have ". . . one-third the number of office-based physicians and one-twentieth the number of hospital-based physicians available to serve children as in the New York metropolitan area where the per capita income is two-thirds again as high as that of the rural South."[29]

When the question of task delegation is raised, regional variations are not nearly as clear. If you consider the delegation of clerical and technical office tasks, there does seem to be some regional variation, as reported by these same AAP pediatricians. The northeastern United States appears the most conservative region in the country regarding its physicians' willingness to delegate these clerical and technical tasks, even though this region has the greatest availability of health manpower.[30] Interestingly, the West, which is that region most willing to delegate these types of tasks, has significantly less health manpower resources available to it than does the Northeast.[31] However, when the more patient-oriented-task delegation (such as well-child care, history taking, or parental counseling) is considered, there is presently very little meaningful delegation, regardless of region.[32] It would appear that nonphysician health care professionals have a significant way to go before exercising independent functioning in the provision of many aspects of primary patient care.

Specialty Distribution within Professions

It is an acknowledged fact that there has been a marked increase in the number of specialists relative to primary care physicians (general practitioners, internists, and pediatricians). In 1972, it was estimated that of the 10,000 June graduates from the 108 U.S. medical schools, only 10 percent had chosen to enter general or family practice, 80 percent had chosen specialty practice while another 10 percent planned to enter academia or research.[33] This move toward specialization has left many patients without ready access to a family physician; specialists deal mainly with referrals from other physicians (initially often a generalist), which results in many people having no access to the bulk of physicians. Additionally, this current distribution has led to an inefficient use of other segments of the health system such as emergency room facilities.

Specialization, of course, is not viewed, nor need it be, entirely negatively. One author sees "the increasing degree of specialization of health manpower, either within a health occupation or in the form of new health occupations as the direct result of improvement in utilization practices."[34] Most frequently, according to this same writer, specialization is said to stem from the increase in scientific knowledge, thereby compelling practitioners to limit themselves to an increasingly smaller portion of health service. This interpretation views specialization as a defensive posture whereby the physician, in an effort to cope with increasing knowledge, retreats to a more circumscribed expertise. Dale Hiestand argues differently: he views specialization as the source of increased knowledge, not the result:

> With limited practice, they [physicians] gained increased skill and productivity through deeper explorations into particular disease entities and medical techniques. . . . More importantly . . . [specialization] leads to higher quality and an increased supply of services, since the specialist can usually handle a given problem better and in less time than a less skilled practitioner.[35]

Both these views of specialization can be used, and have been used, to help justify the introduction of new types of health professionals of which the PA is a good example. This new professional may be seen as providing access to the health system to those in need of primary care. However, they are as easily envisioned as instrumental in providing a means by which the skills of specialists can be used with greater economy—for consultation, for example.

Utilization

Utilization is concerned with how effectively and efficiently the health system exploits the talents of available manpower. "Changes in utilization practices may partially convert the demand for manpower from occupations which are in short supply to those in which manpower can be more readily obtained."[36] One of the most crucial variables in relationship to utilization is the nature of the education provided health workers. Utilization practices should reflect—and be reflected by—

health manpower educational programs. It is frequently the disparity between the content of educational programs in the health professions and the actual practice of these professionals that leads to discontent, high turnover rates, early retirements, and so on, and thus compounds problems stemming from shortages of health workers.

Currently, the nursing profession provides an example of a poor mesh between training and utilization practices as shown by several studies. One recent finding of the National Commission for the Study of Nursing and Nursing Education demonstrates the disparity between nursing education and practice, which accompanied a second disparity between what motivated individuals to enter nursing and the reward system within that profession. With regard to the latter incongruity, it was discovered that many persons were attracted to nursing because of a desire for direct patient care while promotion within the profession usually entailed movement away from direct patient care.[37] Consequently, it is apparent that utilization practices can not only affect the productivity, effectiveness, and efficiency of health care delivery, but also the retention rate of practitioners.

Productivity

There can scarcely be a more important goal than the increase of productivity in order to better serve the health of the nation, but obviously there can be various definitions of what one means by increasing health care productivity. Should the emphasis be placed upon increasing quantitative or qualitative productivity? Perhaps, it is best to attempt both? Various studies have defined productivity differently. For example, an increase in the number of patients seen by a physician in a given length of time may be considered a measure of increased productivity. Using this criterion, one study of Pediatric Nurse Practitioners (PNPs) showed an increase of 18.8 percent in the productivity of two physicians employing a PNP in their office.[38] Increased productivity may be said to be achieved when a larger volume of output can be obtained from a given amount of resources, while holding quality of care constant. Increased productivity may also be achieved when the same volume of output is obtained from the same resources, but output becomes of better quality; for example, additional services not previously available (such as home visits) are offered.

There are essentially three means available to achieve increased productivity.[39] Professionals can apply more or different facilities, equipment, and materials that may increase the productivity of existing health manpower. Examples of such measures to augment productivity may include the use of computerized health information systems, using disposable implements (for example, syringes), and locating physicians' offices closer to hospitals. The organization and scale of health delivery may also lead to increasing the productivity of existing health manpower. For example, several authors have suggested that group practice should lead to an increase of the productivity of physicians. A third method, and perhaps the most interesting (at least for our concerns), is the transfer of functions or tasks from more highly skilled health professionals to the lesser skilled in order to increase the effective output of the former. The dental profession has, particularly within the last decade, shown how they have substantially increased productivity through the use of better equipment and ancillary personnel, such as dental hygienists.[40]

Transfer of function might be accomplished in one of three ways. Tasks might be shifted upward if they could be performed more efficiently by more highly skilled personnel. Specialists performing very skilled work within circumscribed boundaries might provide an example of this type of transfer, provided that it was determined this task could be accomplished more efficiently at the higher level; that is, that it would create less cost per unit output for similar or improved quality and quantity of work. Tasks could remain at the same level, but workers could be given additional training so that their performance would become more efficient (less cost) or more effective (better quality)—or both. The use of the NP might provide a good example of this potential type of transfer. Lastly, tasks could be shifted downward to less highly skilled and lower paid workers if quality and quantity of service could be maintained. The transfer of diagnostic tasks from a physician to his PA might serve as an example of such a transfer.

Any such transfer of function necessitates prior task analysis in order to record the time various workers spend doing different tasks, so as to isolate time ill spent on tasks that could be better performed by other members of the health team. A number of studies conducted in this area have been initiated in order to assess the introduction of two new health professionals to the health care system: the PA and the NP. Several of these studies are discussed in Chapter 4. The local case study reported in Chapter 6 considers the acceptance and appropriateness of one such transfer—that of certain obstetrical tasks to obstetrical PAs. How much would this increase productivity, and what would be the patients' response?

Demand and Supply Factors

Demand

The demand for health manpower* is a derived demand. It stems from the demand for health care that comprises diverse services

*This discussion closely follows Irene Butter, "Health Manpower Research: A Survey," Inquiry 4, no. 4 (December 1967): 6-7

provided by the combined efforts of many health workers together with nonlabor inputs such as capital, equipment, or facilities. The requirement for any particular category of health service is derived from three factors: (1) the demand for health care services (both volume and composition); (2) the setting (the technical, organizational, and institutional processes that together provide health services); and (3) the productivity—the average volume of services that is or will be rendered per man hour in each of the health professions; that is, each health profession's capacity to meet demand.

The demand for health care services may also be viewed as the combined effect of various demographic, socioeconomic, and political factors, as was alluded to in Chapter 1. Demographic factors include population size and density, age distribution, sex ratio, and corresponding patterns of diseases themselves. Socioeconomic aspects, such as the degree of urbanization, play on such things as the rates of mental disturbances and environmental pollution. Upper income groups have, for example, a greater marginal propensity to consume and thereby may demand certain types of health care. Industrialization is closely tied to the incidence of such diseases as silicosis. Higher educational attainment correlates with the ability to use the health system, particularly for preventive care. Such groups are also more likely to be more politicized with regard to health care and to push for such things as more effective private and government health insurance. The social philosophy of an incumbent government obviously affects demand. Is access to adequate health care the right of all citizens? Such programs as Medicare and Medicaid reflect a movement in such a direction. Closely aligned with this is the question of whether or not persons of political influence elect to view demand primarily in an economic or noneconomic sense. The former, of course, emphasizes the ability to pay and relies upon the marketplace to distribute services. The philosophy of allocating health services according to one's ability to pay (rather than adopting a more normative criterion) stands as an obstacle to a rational utilization of health services: income and not medical need too often determines if one sees an optometrist or opthalmologist, a podiatrist or orthopedist.

Supply

In concluding, some of the factors affecting recruitment and retention of health workers can be briefly mentioned—all of which could be critical factors in determining the supply of newly emerging health professionals. Without question, the economic reward (or enticement) offered by the position is an important variable, particularly as viewed from the standpoint of rate of return on investment made in training or value of lifetime earnings. However, nonmonetary factors are not to be ignored in the development of effective recruitment. Such attributes of a profession as prestige, personal challenge, and an opportunity to serve are of considerable importance. The capacity and distribution of training programs, as well as the availability of stipends, are highly relevant factors, as is the dissemination of information concerning the profession. Licensure requirement is another example of a variable which not only can restrict entry, but may also reduce career mobility and inhibit lateral and vertical mobility; thus, recruitment and retention may be adversely affected in an occupation requiring licensure.

Attrition rates experienced during professional training have an obvious effect on supply of different types of health workers. For example, currently attrition in nursing schools is quite high, whereas in medical schools it is comparatively low. This is undoubtedly partially due to recruitment: medical schools have rather stringent entrance requirements (only one-third to one-half of the applicants are admitted); however, nursing schools (particularly diploma programs) do not operate at full capacity.

The net supply (retention) of professional health workers—especially nonphysicians—is crucially affected by another three factors: post-training attrition due to nonemployment, early retirement, and the rate of return of inactive workers. These factors are affected by a number of closely linked variables including: (1) the closeness of fit between workers' education and their practice; (2) the attractiveness of the job (setting, hours, and so on); (3) potential for career development; (4) geographic and occupational mobility; and (5) the existence and nature of reentry enticements. For example, approximately one-quarter of professional nurses maintain their license, another one-fourth maintain a license but do not practice, while another 15 percent work only part time.[41]

CONCLUDING REMARKS

The preceding pages briefly discussed some of the behavioral science literature most relevant to understanding changes occurring within the U.S. health delivery system. This should have particular applicability for forthcoming research, investigating innovations in health manpower, such as the introduction of the PA and NP. It is hoped that this discussion will be useful for those interested in designing research generated by and contributing to these rich theoretical traditions.

With reference to the author's research, this selected review of the literature served a twofold purpose. First, it drew together theoretical insights from different traditions in order to provide a sound basis for research on the PA. Second, the literature identified general issue areas likely to be of major concern to those parties affected by the entry of a new health provider into the present system. These broader issue areas were then recast to reflect substantive concerns of the PA. For example, the more general issue area of role conflict (with its well-established body of associated theory) could then be particularized into questions examining the role relationship between the nurse and the PA. In this manner, the survey instruments were designed. The results of the national and local surveys (integrated with a substantial amount of selected PA literature) provide the focus for the following three chapters.

NOTES

1. Everett M. Rogers and F. Floyd Shoemaker, Communication of Innovations: A Cross-Cultural Approach (New York: The Free Press, 1971), p. 19.
2. Ibid., pp. 62-64.
3. Ibid., pp. 138-139.
4. Ibid., pp. 145-148.
5. Ibid., p. 148.
6. Ibid., p. 189.
7. Ibid., p. 155.
8. Ibid., pp. 185-191.
9. Herbert F. Lionberger, Adoption of New Ideas and Practices (Ames, Iowa: Iowa State University Press, 1960), p. 68.
10. Ibid., pp. 82-83.
11. Ibid., p. 97.
12. Lewis A. Coser, The Functions of Social Conflict (New York: The Free Press, 1956), p. 153.
13. Melvin L. DeFleur, William V. D'Antonio, and Lois B. DeFleur, Sociology: Man in Society (Glenview, Ill.: Scott Foresman, 1971), p. 48.
14. Elliott A. Krause, The Sociology of Occupations (Boston: Little, Brown, 1971), p. 141.
15. Ibid., p. 146.
16. Irene Butter, "Health Manpower Research: A Survey," Inquiry 4, no. 4 (December 1967): 6-7.
17. Ibid., p. 8.
18. Ibid., p. 31.
19. Surgeon General's Consultant Group on Medical Education, Physicians for a Growing America (Washington, D.C.: U.S. Government Printing Office, 1959), cited in W. Lee Hanson, "An Appraisal of Physician Manpower Projections," Inquiry 7, no. 1 (March 1970): 106.
20. W. Lee Hanson, "An Appraisal of Physician Manpower Projections," Inquiry 7, no. 1 (March 1970): 110.
21. Gaston W. Rimlinger and Henry B. Steele, "An Economic Interpretation of the Spatial Distributions of Physicians in the U.S.," The Southern Economics Journal 30, no. 1 (July 1963), cited in Butter, op. cit., p. 32.

22. Eli Ginzberg with Miriam Ostow, Men, Money and Medicine (New York: Columbia University Press, 1969), p. 113.

23. Butter, op. cit., p. 10.

24. National Commission for the Study of Nursing and Nursing Education, "Nurse Clinician and Physician's Assistant: The Relationship Between Two Emerging Practitioner Concepts," Rochester, New York: The Commission, 1971.

25. Butter, op. cit., p. 10.

26. Ibid., pp. 6-7.

27. Alfred Yankauer, John P. Connelly, Priscilla Andrews, and Jacob J. Feldman, "The Practice of Nursing in Pediatric Offices—Challenge and Opportunity," New England Journal of Medicine 282 (April 1970): 844.

28. Ibid., p. 846.

29. Alfred Yankauer, John P. Connelly, and Jacob J. Feldman, "Physician Productivity in the Delivery of Ambulatory Care: Some Findings from a Survey of Pediatricians," Medical Care 8, no. 1 (January-February 1970): 36.

30. Yankauer, Connelly, Andrews, and Feldman, op. cit., p. 844.

31. Ibid.

32. Ibid., p. 845.

33. Malcolm C. Todd, "Medical Manpower and the Emergence of New Professions," Texas Medicine 68, no. 10 (October 1972): 60.

34. Dale L. Hiestand, "Research into Manpower for Health Service," Milbank Memorial Fund Quarterly 44, no. 4 (October 1966): 171.

35. Ibid., pp. 171-172.

36. Ibid., p. 167.

37. National Commission for the Study of Nursing and Nursing Education, op. cit.

38. Donald W. Schiff, Charles H. Frazer, and Heather L. Walters, "The Pediatric Nurse Practitioner in the Office of Pediatricians in Private Practice," Pediatrics 44, no. 1 (July 1969): 65.

39. Butter, op. cit., p. 29.

40. Jeffrey H. Weiss, "A Job Classification Scheme for Health Manpower," Health Services Report 3, no. 1 (Spring 1968): 44-64.

41. National Commission for the Study of Nursing and Nursing Education, op. cit.

CHAPTER

4

THE STATUS OF THE PA: SELECTED EARLY PA LITERATURE AND A NATIONAL SURVEY OF EARLY PA PROGRAMS

INITIAL DEVELOPMENT OF A CONCEPT

In 1961, Charles L. Hudson suggested the creation of two new groups of assistants to physicians to be drawn from nonmedical, nonnursing personnel.[1] The first was to be an on-the-job trained medical assistant who would be responsible for many of the highly skilled but technical medical tasks assumed by physicians; for example, performing lumbar punctures. Although such an assistant would have significant technical skill, he would not be expected to exercise medical judgment; his role would be clearly delineated by the physician-employer who would consequently be legally responsible for the actions of his assistant.[2] The similarities between this first type of assistant suggested by Hudson in 1961 and the assistant designated as "Type C" in 1970 by the National Academy of Sciences are easily noted.

Hudson felt that a second type of assistant would be even more desirable; these "externes" would be ". . .assistants with special training, intermediate between that of the technician and that of the doctor, who could not only handle many technical procedures. . .but could also take some degree of medical responsibility."[3] Externes would be educated in a college program of two to three years duration with appropriate additional clinical training. Although very similar to the "Type A" physician's assistant (PA) of the late 1960s, Hudson's concept of an externe was closely tied to the hospital. In fact, the primary impetus for both of Hudson's assistants was a reaction to the shortage of medical-professional personnel to aid the physician in his expanding and time-consuming hospital practice, thus allowing the physician to devote more time to his community practice. Although the assistant was to be supervised by a physician, Hudson felt that it would be the hospital that would contemplate his employment.[4]

It is worth noting some of the potential objections Hudson foresaw to the introduction of the externe, as many of these same issues were subsequently debated in the 1960-to-early-1970 PA literature. Objections would center on problems of recruitment, on an inability to establish a satisfactory interposition for the PA between medicine and nursing, on issues of acceptability, particularly by nurses and by patients, and finally, on assertions that no new group was needed to assist the medical field as the goals of nursing could be redefined as part medicine and part nursing.[5] Hudson, however, was sensitive to the goals of nursing—and how they differed from those of medicine. He felt that

> . . . nursing would not find the proposal of a medicine-nursing hybrid consistent with their present goals for nurse education. . . . It would seem incautious to presume that nurses and nursing should be the principal field for the recruitment of externes or their counterparts, without at least the endorsement of the nursing profession.[6]

Interestingly, it was just such unilateral presumption by the American Medical Association (AMA) in 1970 that evoked a sharp rebuke from the American Nurses' Association (ANA).

It was in late 1964 that Hudson's concept of an externe began to take shape. Discovering that physicians were simply too busy to attend a series of planned postgraduate seminars, Eugene Stead, M.D., then professor and chairman of the Department of Medicine at Duke University, began to lay the foundation for what was to be the first physician's assistant training program in the United States. In order to facilitate more efficient utilization of existing physicians and nurses, Stead felt that many highly technical, though repetitive and time-consuming, tasks could be delegated to properly trained medical assistants. In February 1965, this proposed new health provider was defined in a report of Duke's Ad Hoc Committee to the 62nd Annual Congress on Medical Education:

> The physician's assistant is seen as a new category within the structure of the health field designed to provide a career opportunity for men functioning under the direction of doctors with greater capabilities and growth potential than informally trained technicians.[7]

As initially designed, the Duke program recruited primarily males (more career oriented), who were ex-military corpsmen (possessed prior health education and experience), and who were not nurses (would not aggravate the nursing shortage).[8] A pilot program began in 1965 with the selection of four ex-military corpsmen who were then studied as they progressed through the program as a basis for continuing curriculum development and evaluation. A certificate, not a degree, was awarded at the completion of the program.

ISSUES OF CONSEQUENCE

Introducing a new health professional into the health field was bound to generate comment—both positive and negative. The medical profession was undecided about the potential use of this new assistant—the idea of someone not trained as a physician participating in a limited practice of medicine was one to be subjected to the utmost scrutiny. The relationship between nursing and this new profession "somewhere between nursing and medicine" was yet to be established. Would the patient accept this new health provider or would he be considered the purveyor of second-class medicine to be tolerated only by the poor or medically disadvantaged? What would be the legal status of this new practitioner? What effect, if any, would the PA have on the spiraling costs of medical care?

In late 1970, none of these broader issues had been definitively resolved although a number of preliminary studies had been completed that had provided valuable insights. In addition, many more basic issues were still the focus of debate. How was the PA to be defined? Should the PA be a specialist or a generalist? What would be the appropriate content and setting of a program purporting to educate PAs? How was the functional role of the PA to be defined? Where should recruits for PA programs be sought? Where had the initial graduates of PA programs been placed? Had they been well accepted?

In an attempt to begin to answer these types of questions, the first two approaches to an exploratory study were combined; that is, a more extensive literature review was undertaken and combined with the results of the author's 1970 national survey of both the operative and planned PA programs previously identified. (See Chapter 2.)

TOWARD A DEFINITION OF THE PHYSICIAN'S ASSISTANT

When first coined by Duke University, the term physician's assistant (PA) was intended to be a label for new health professionals who were trained by physicians, worked for physicians, were responsible to physicians, and were capable of assuming many tasks and functions which were traditionally performed by physicians. The PA was not intended to be a "super-technician" or a "super-nurse;" he was simply to be an assistant to the physician.[9]

In the five years that had passed since the Duke program began, the term PA had become fairly widespread in use. A variety of programs began and, although all did not define the PA in an identical fashion, were subsumed under the umbrella term of PA. In May 1970, the National Academy of Sciences published a report entitled, "New Members of the Physician's Health Team: Physician's Assistants."[10] Acknowledging the great variety of functions to be potentially delegated to PAs, the diverse circumstances in which they would work, and the different types and levels of skill required, the concept of the PA was divided into three categories: Type A, Type B, and Type C physician's assistants.[11] Since these definitions have already been presented earlier in the text, they do not need reiteration; however, the important point to stress is that great flexibility existed, and continues to be encouraged, in defining the PA. Although in many instances this lack of precise definition has proven to be an asset (that is, in allowing broad latitude in defining scope of appropriate functions), it has also been a source of much confusion. Specifically, much confusion (and consternation) has resulted from the initial inclusion of nurse practitioner programs in lists of PA programs.[12] (While acknowledging this confusion, the author still chose to include several NP programs in her surveys; where applicable, similarities and differences between the NP and the nonnurse-PA were reflected in the analysis of the data.*)

Each of the training programs in the author's 1970 national survey was asked to define the term PA within the context of its own program. Upon reviewing the answers, major similarities and differences became apparent. The vast majority of the programs included some equivalent of the phrase: the physician's assistant is to work with and under the supervision of a physician. There were two notable differences in the programs' interpretations of how this requirement should be put into operation. Many felt that it meant that there must be a direct one-to-one relationship between an employing physician and his employee, the PA. As one program director stated, "The apostrophe in physician's assistant makes the phrase singularly possessive and not plurally permissive."[13] However, this interpretation did not, in all cases,

---

*Several NP programs were included in the author's 1970 national survey of PA programs; that is, of the 31 PA programs in the study, 11 could be classified as NP programs. The text reflects instances where NP program responses to specific questions differed substantially from those of nonnurse-PA programs. In the author's 1973 restudy of PA programs, the entire original national sample was recontacted, including the NP programs. However, in the ensuing two or three years, there had been a rather definitive separation of the two types of programs; therefore, the responses of the two types of programs were analyzed separately and their uniqueness was discussed.

mean that the PA could not be employed in a group practice. In such instances, the PA might be responsible to different members of the group at different times of the day or week, although at all times ". . . all acts of these new health workers would, for each such act, be under the direct orders and control of a specific individual physician."[14]

There was little agreement among the programs in their interpretations of the phrase "under the supervision of the physician." For some it meant that the PA would only be allowed to function in the physician's office when the physician was also present. Others felt that the availability of telephone communication between the PA and his physician-employer constituted sufficient supervision. Some felt strongly that all procedures of the PA should be subject to direct review of the supervising physician while others felt that "review as needed" was adequate. A California legal-medicine foundation made the following caution with regard to the interpretation of "under the supervision of a physician:"

> If "health care tasks" are to be delegated and the PA may perform "medical services," there is little doubt that he will be practicing medicine within the legal meaning of that phrase. . . . "Under the supervision" of the physician cannot mean under his direct and immediate guidance; that is, the physician's presence at all times in the room where the PA carries out medical tasks. . . the well trained and reliable PA in whom the physician has complete confidence probably will be carrying out a variety of medical tasks (that is, tasks which a physician ordinarily accomplishes and not a nurse) independently. . . . [Where negligence becomes a concern] the central question concerns the standard of care issue.[15]

The standard of care issue is only one of many legal issues surrounding the use of the PA that must be resolved if the PA is to be widely accepted and efficiently utilized. Further consideration will be given these legal issues later in the chapter.

Another program was more optimistic about the potential for use of a PA in situations which did not require immediate physical supervision by the physician-employer.

> In today's world of modern and sophisticated communications devices, it is possible for physicians to exercise "responsible supervision" over paramedics with great latitude as to the active distance between them rather than being confined to "direct supervision," which has the connotation of being at his elbow.[16]

At least six states have shown agreement with this position by provisions, within their PA-related legislation, to qualify the degree of supervision and control needed between the PA and his physician-employer. Laws in Arkansas, Florida, Iowa, New York, Oklahoma, and Utah stipulate that supervision and control need not mean the direct or permanent presence of the supervising physician at the PA's site of activity.[17]

The vast majority of the programs, when defining the PA, stressed the PA's "physician dependent" role. Even those programs training Type A PAs (those PAs who can exercise a limited degree of independent medical judgment) stressed the physician dependency of their assistants. PAs are trained as ". . . dependent assistants, working with and responsible to a physician. They do not write prescriptions, make diagnosis, or initiate treatment."[18] Although again stressing the dependency of the PA role, one PA program had taken the necessary steps to legitimize the ability of their graduates to, within predetermined limits, diagnose, counsel, and prescribe in both health and illness.[19] Another program felt that, although the PA was a true "associate" of the physician, he ". . . could function only as an agent of the physician in a clearly delineated set of activities."[20]

Programs which prepare nurses for an expanded role emphasized that their graduates, as nurses and thus independent professionals in their own right, should make independent nursing judgments. Although assuming some of the physician's traditional tasks, the nursing component (for example, caring, nurturing, teaching) of the NP role was to be stressed. While the NP would always

> . . . serve under the general supervision of a physician. . . he may not always be physically present. Within this framework, these nurses are frequently called upon to make independent nursing judgments based on previous education and experience and enhanced by the advanced preparation which they receive in the program.[21]

As such, NP programs emphasized that they were not training assistants but rather, they were educating nurse associates or nurse practitioners. They stressed the collaborative relationship that should exist between these professionals and the physician with whom they work. Patient care should be a shared responsibility between the nurse practitioner, the physician, and other members of the health team. "Physicians and nurses can and should work together to determine which of them can best assume responsibility for a particular aspect of a patient's therapeutic regime."[22] Often this involves a realignment of functions between medicine and nursing.

That the skills of nursing and medicine are different and that these differences are (and should be) reflected in the definition of the NP and PA roles, respectively, was noted in a succinct fashion in at least one PA program. "Nursing has evolved into a professional arena of its own, serving the patient in such a way as to enhance his comfort, speed his recovery, and enable him to live with his limitations."[23]

Therefore, because of nursing's unique competence, the NP might be better equipped than a nonnurse PA to function in settings characterized by low population densities, poor transportation, and a relative absence of physicians; the NP could then be considered as an ". . . independent assistant who functions with a degree of autonomy, limited usually by the complexity of the patient's problem which the worker himself must evaluate."[24] This is in contrast to the PA who functions most effectively where there is a shortage of physicians but where the population served is generally well educated and transportation to health facilities is efficient. The PA is then defined as a

> . . . dependent health care worker, working under direct supervision of the physician, but performing tasks once done by the physician. . . . He has definite limitations, the most constraining being that he can only function when the physician is able to readily see the patient, evaluate the assistant's findings, give him guidance, and make decisions.[25]

It should be noted that one could endorse the above distinction between NPs and PAs without denying the ability of either health professional to function in settings physically removed from the physician-employer. Geographic separation and functional independence are two separate issues. If one accepted such a difference between a NP and a PA, the NP would enjoy both geographic separation and at least some functional independence while the PA might be geographically separated from his physician-employer, although he would still be a functionally dependent health provider.

Several programs included references in their definitions of a PA to the settings in which they felt the PA should function. In general, most programs felt that the PA could work in both the hospital and the office practice of a physician as long as he was working under the supervision of his physician-employer. Only one program specifically mentioned that their concept of a PA was of one who ". . . may not be employed by a hospital or lay group."[26] Some hospitals have not allowed PAs to write orders or function in their full capacity in a hospital setting, even when the PA is functioning only as an agent of his physician-employer. As the hospital becomes more and more the focus of health care in the United States, the PA, if he is to become a viable member of the health team, must be able to function within the hospital. As Duke University's program stated:

> There is nothing to preclude the use of physician's assistants in the hospital setting as indicated by the status of the following three issues relating to such use as trained physician's assistants. First, existing legislation in most states is compatible with utilizing physician's assistants in the hospital setting so long as the assistant is under the super-

vision of a physician and functions within the limiting legal framework. Second, the current position of the Joint Commission on Hospital Accreditation is compatible with the use of physician's assistants in the hospital setting. So far as is known, no health-related professional organization has taken any stand in opposition to this issue. Third, in all existing situations, the issue of professional liability coverage has created no difficulty for the hospital, the physician, or the physician's assistant.[27]

The above 1970 position, held by Duke's PA program on the need for, and capability of, the PA to function within the hospital is in keeping with Hudson's original position on the appropriate work setting for his externe. However, contrary to Hudson's position, Duke has stated that the PA is not intended to be an institutional employee. His role in the hospital would be supervised and directed by his physician-employer. In addition, ". . . if an assistant is to function in a hospital, he must be granted limited staff privileges and must participate as a member of the institution's medical staff."[28] This position is congruent with a statement on the role of the PA in the hospital adopted by the American Hospital Association (AHA) early in 1971. The AHA would apply the PA label ". . . only to individuals who work full time for a physician in the performance of tasks assigned by that physician, whether they are employed by the physician or by the hospital."[29] Although a PA, supervised by a physician, may function within a hospital, his use would be subject to strict professional review by the medical staff regarding the PA's training, experience, and specific task capability. Hospital bylaws would need to be changed to allow the granting of limited staff privileges to qualified PAs; guidelines for the needed changes were issued in 1971 by the Joint Commission on Accreditation of Hospitals.[30]

By 1972, only four states (New York, Florida, Oklahoma, and West Virginia) had provided the legal stimulus, within their PA-related legislation, to encourage the hospital to incorporate the assistant into its organizational setting.[31] That the PA has a legitimate role in all facets of his physician-employer's practice, including the hospital, is generally accepted. However, although several important steps had been taken to encourage such use, the issue was by no means resolved by mid-1972.

PRIMARY CARE PROVIDER OR SPECIALIST?

What type of PA were the programs predominantly educating in 1970? Were generalists being trained to provide primary care or were the majority of the programs training specialists in order to complement the general trend in medicine toward specialization? Of the 31 programs whose responses were included in the 1970 national survey, 11 emphasized the training of generalists—those who would be concerned with providing primary care. Eleven were limited to the pediatrics specialty; since a pediatrician is often considered a child's general practitioner, perhaps these programs can be classified between those programs which prepare generalists and those which prepare specialists. Thirteen programs prepared types of PAs who were oriented toward a particular specialty such as anesthesia, pathology, surgery, coronary care, and ophthalmology. (The number exceeds the total of programs since some programs train both specialists and generalists.)

Duke's PA program, the forerunner in the PA movement, has consistently emphasized ". . . the area of general medicine, because the most evident need was help for the first-line, community-based physician."[32] However, responding to specialists' demands, the program was gradually expanded to include several specialty and subspecialty options. The evident need for the generalist was stressed in a recent book by Rashi Fein entitled <u>The Doctor Shortage: An Economic Diagnosis</u>. In 1931, only 17 percent of the physicians in private practice considered themselves specialists; by 1965, 64 percent considered themselves to be engaged in specialty practice.[33] Although the last few years have seen a small resurgence of interest in community practice (as witnessed by the rise of a "new specialty" called family practice), the trend toward a higher percentage of pure specialists continues. According to one government sponsored survey, as of 1967 over 97 percent of medical students on a national basis were planning to go into specialty practice.[34]

Obviously, the rise in the number of specialists has been associated with a concurrent decline in the number of general practitioners. What are the implications for patient care of this trend? "The physician in general practice performed some functions that now go largely unfulfilled. He offered primary care. . . [he was] the family's doctor."[35] If the PA concept is an attempt to expand the availability of primary medical care and to provide more and better access to high quality care for more people, with an emphasis on those who are most severely medically disadvantaged (for example, the poor, rural residents, the elderly), the functions now largely unfulfilled due to a scarcity of general practitioners should logically be satisfied.[36] However, if the PA is encouraged to become too specialty-oriented and thus complements the specialty maldistribution that presently exists, this approach toward a partial resolution of the health manpower shortage may prove ineffectual. If this occurs, one cannot blame the PA. In a specialty-dominated medical marketplace, the specialty-trained PA may find his skills more saleable than those of his generalist counterpart. However, he runs the risk of built-in obsolescence if his skills become too narrowly circumscribed and tailored to meet today's technological specialty needs.

Rashi Fein further illustrates that the decline in general practitioners is also associated with an increasing geographic maldistribution in medical service availability. "The more specialized the physician, the less likely it will be that some areas will be adequately served—either in total numbers or in terms of the mix of physicians."[37] Those who view the health manpower crisis as one of distribution, and not simply of numbers, would advance the following question: "How will overlapping this distorted pattern of distribution with a parallel distribution of physician's assistants produce meaningful advantages for medically deprived persons and areas?"[38] This question is particularly relevant if the PA is only allowed to practice in close proximity to his physician-employer or is not encouraged or is not permitted to be primarily employed by health agencies (for example, hospitals, neighborhood health centers, public health departments), where he might be deployed in geographic areas most in need of accessible primary health care.

DEVELOPMENT OF A JOB DESCRIPTION FOR THE PA

In the 1970 national survey, the programs were asked how they had developed an appropriate job description for each of the various types of PAs being trained. Only one program specifically stated that they had used the guidelines suggested by the National Academy of Sciences' definition of a Type A physician's assistant.[39] The pediatric nurse practitioner programs had relied heavily upon guidelines developed by a Joint Committee of the American Nurses' Association and the American Academy of Pediatrics (AAP) to develop their job descriptions; building upon a firm foundation of nursing theory and skills, the PNP job description extended the nursing role to include skills which are traditionally in the area of the physician-pediatrician; the skills selected for delegation to the PNP were based on prior task analyses and interdisciplinary conferences.

Approximately six of the 31 programs emphasized the need for task analysis of the specialist or general practitioner with whom the PA was to work. Some of the specialty-oriented programs had conducted extensive analyses of their specialist-physicians; in particular, there was a time-motion study of pediatricians[40] and a task analysis of anesthesiologists.[41] One program looked intensively at the jobs that needed to be done and then trained people to do those particular jobs;[42] another looked at the health needs of a particular patient group (for example, men at sea) and developed job descriptions accordingly;[43] still another conducted an attitude study of potential patients to determine what tasks performed by a PA would be acceptable to those patients.[44] Several programs trained PAs in a generalist core curriculum; specific job descriptions were then expected to be individually developed by the individual PA in collaboration with his physician-employer.[45]

Two programs approached the task of job description in a somewhat unique and (in the author's opinion) particularly thorough manner. The two approaches were nearly diametrically opposed. The first program recruited several students (in this instance, medical corpsmen) and taught them on a one-to-one basis over several years. As the students progressed through the, at first, informal program, they were studied carefully in order to determine how much and how fast they could learn and what types of procedures they could satisfactorily perform.[46] The second program employed a more academic approach, in contrast to the former more pragmatic approach, to the development of a job description. An interdisciplinary advisory council was constituted that involved representatives from all relevant academic departments of the college (sociology, allied health sciences, nursing, and medicine), members of the college's administration, members of the medical staff of the local college-affiliated hospital, and representatives of the major medical and nursing professional organizations in the state. From this council emerged five broad categories of activities with which the PA would be involved. These broad categories were then broken down into the more detailed tasks which the PA could be expected to do in each of two settings: the hospital or the office and clinic.[47]

Most programs did not wish tc delineate detailed lists of tasks which the PA could do under the supervision of his physician-employer. To rigidly specify what the PA could or could not do was felt to place undue restrictions on his employer and would possibly prevent needed flexibility for the development of the new role. However, programs did prepare graduates for certain common competencies in the following types of tasks: medical and family history; comprehensive physical examinations; screening tests (for example, for visual or hearing disorders or routine neurological tests); routine laboratory tests (such as blood counts, urinalysis, tests of basal metabolic rates); collection of specimens (for such purposes as gastric analysis or blood studies); cast application and traction adjustment; suturing of minor lacerations; routine dressing changes; and starting and regulating intravenous treatments. Most PAs were to make rounds with their physicians or supplement rounds or both to explain treatments and procedures to patients, allay apprehensions, and the like. Some PAs, who were to be employed primarily in office practices, were given some training in clerical and administrative tasks; one program mentioned that the PA could be responsible for the overall management of the physician's office. As one program explained, the PA would be ". . . an observer and a fact finder. Interpretation of facts, and decisions regarding treatment were not proposed as his province."[48]

Although many of the specific technical tasks to be delegated to the nonnurse PA were similar to those which were to be included in the competency of the NP, there were certain notable differences—in emphasis as well as in substance. As the nonnurse PA, the NP was to be proficient in taking a medical and social history (with special emphasis on the careful sequential pinpointing of signs and symptoms), conducting a comprehensive physical examination (including a complete developmental assessment), and performing laboratory tests (such as cultures, urinalysis, and blood counts). In addition to the delegation of these more medical and technical tasks, the NP was to expand upon the nursing component of her role. This was evident in at least two respects: (1) the emphasis in the NP role was on health as opposed to being upon disease; many of her tasks were consequently focused on promoting health maintenance, on patient teaching, counseling, and the provision of anticipatory guidance; and (2) although the NP would be involved in the management of illness, an emphasis was placed on the psychosocial aspects of such management as well as the more traditional medical aspects; that is, an emphasis was placed on caring for the patient as an individual and as a member of a community and on promoting both physical and mental comfort by nursing as well as medical interventions. This is not to say that the nonnurse PA was not concerned with health maintenance or with the psychosocial aspects of health care; rather, the NP role was clearly more oriented toward these facets of care. Although many of the tasks delegated were similar, the nonnurse PA was educated to adopted the "mind-set of the physician"[49] whereas the NP was expected to expand upon her nursing role as well as receive a greater delegation of medical tasks.

RECRUITMENT SOURCES FOR THE PA ROLE

Another issue considered in the 1970 national survey of PA programs was that of recruitment: specifically, what would be appropriate manpower sources from which the PA could and should be recruited? Since the programs varied substantially in their definitions of the PA and in the jobs these professionals were to fulfill, it was assumed that opinions regarding proper recruitment sources would also vary greatly. In addition to eliciting what recruitment source each program felt to be the right one, an attempt was made to ascertain why the particular choice had been made.

The Nurse as a Recruitment Source

The major recruitment sources preferred by the programs were registered nurses (RNs) and ex-military medical corpsmen. In addition to the ten NP programs in the survey, two of the nonnurse PA programs mentioned the RN as one of their preferred types of recruits. Of the ten NP programs, four recruited only RNs with a baccalaureate degree and one recruited only RNs working within their particular hospital.

One of the programs, recruiting RNs for further training as PNPs (Pediatric Nurse Practioners) aptly summarized the reasons for their particular recruitment choice; their reasons are indicative of the reasons cited by the other programs:

> a. She [the nurse] has always been held in high regard by the public; therefore, medical care and advice given by the nurse will most likely be accepted by the parents and patients. . . . [In addition]. . . Many nurses with basic knowledge and skills live in rural areas where they have established homes and families. . .
>
> b. Physicians and nurses have traditionally worked together as the two major professions providing care. This working together has not always been as coprofessionals sharing the responsibilities involved in meeting health care needs. Physicians have expressed increased willingness to place confidence and responsibility in the nurse as a collaborative colleague while professional nursing education is increasing its preparation in problem solving and decision making . . .
>
> c. Current State Nurse Practice Acts allow wide latitude in services rendered by nurses under the supervision of physicians and for which she has been educationally prepared, so there will be few anticipated legal difficulties . . .
>
> d. Nurses represent the largest active and inactive manpower pool of professionals with the necessary knowledge and experience on which to build those skills required . . .
>
> e. The utilization of nurses in expanded roles in ambulatory care may not be in conflict with the acute nursing shortages in hospitals. A high percentage of the 285, 000 licensed, but currently not practicing, registered nurses in the United States have no desire to return to full or part time hospital nursing. . . 35% of all practicing registered nurses practice outside the hospital setting. . .[50]

The positive attributes of the utilization of RNs (as stated above) may appear to ignore the previously cited statements of the ANA and NLN (see Chapter 1) regarding their reluctance to endorse the use of the RN as a physician's assistant. However, the above statement is essentially a rationale for the use of the nurse as a pediatric nurse associate or practitioner; the job description for this particular type of PA (using the term PA in the generic sense) was developed and endorsed by a joint committee of the ANA and the AAP. However, even with such endorsement, some nursing leaders have not forgotten that

> . . . the concept, the training and the promotion of nurse practitioners appear to have originated with physicians.

> Unfortunately, this, plus semantic difficulty over terms such as task delegation and [the concept of the] physician assuming responsibility for all actions, has caused some nursing leaders to view the nurse practitioner as the physician's assistant [in the narrow sense] and abandoning her identity as a professional nurse.[51]

The two nonnurse PA programs who felt that nurses were appropriate recruits for their programs cited the inadequate utilization of many nurses in both office and hospital practice. The nurses' health and medical knowledge as well as her experience in the health field were highly valued assets which could be put to use in the PA role, adding to the new role and drawing additional skills from it. The remaining PA programs, although admitting the health experience of the nurse would be useful in the PA role, did not favor the nurse being utilized as a PA. Without specifically acknowledging the statement of the ANA and the NLN, some programs felt that the nurse was already in short supply and therefore should not be used for the new role; others felt that the PA's job was too technical and therefore felt that the nurses' nursing skills would be wasted if she functioned primarily as a technician. Still others felt that, since nurses have an exceedingly high turnover rate and a high dropout rate due to the demands of marriage and family responsibilities, perhaps the continuity and stability of the PA role would be threatened by recruiting too many nurses; they felt the desired continuity and stability needed to establish a new profession would be enhanced by recruiting from the broader population and not concentrating on recruits from an existing female-dominated health profession.

The Ex-Military Medical Corpsman as a Recruitment Source

Approximately 12 of the PA programs in the 1970 national survey emphasized the use of ex-military corpsmen as a logical recruitment source for the PA. Essentially, the primary argument for the use of corpsmen was based upon supply and demand; that is, there is a demand for civilian health personnel and there is a supply of ex-military corpsmen having relevant education and experience in the health field. If they are not allowed access into the health field in positions which lend them financial security and personal satisfaction, these veteran corpsmen may be lost to the health field completely. One source estimated that each year approximately 30, 000 medics are discharged from the service; of these, about one-third find their way into civilian health employment; another one-third choose to forget their medical training; the remaining one-third would like to obtain health jobs but are unable to do so.[52] Since it has been estimated that the training of each medic costs the taxpayer up to $25, 000, recruiting ex-medics into PA programs would appear to be an economically sound investment for society.[53]

Although most sources have emphasized the sizeable pool of ex-corpsmen available for potential recruitment into PA programs, some studies have raised some interesting cautions toward a too rapid reliance on this potential source of recruits. What are the characteristics of the ex-medic? Was his service as a medic a voluntary selection or was it decided for him? Upon examining such questions, one study reported that, although sizeable numbers of corpsmen are separated annually from the services, the numbers professing any long term interest in a health career may be considerably less; for example, medical corpsmen are recruited from the ranks of conscientious objectors; as such, they are often better educated than the average recruit, as they are likely to possess some college education if not a B.A. degree. Their prior education may render them overeducated for the civilian level performance of a medical corpsman.[54]

Since there are several PA programs on a baccalaureate or master's level, ex-medics possessing B.A. degrees may still find this a satisfying career; however, a college-educated individual obviously has considerable options; if many ex-medics are in fact college-educated, this would have significant implications for the type of PA programs which should be encouraged. The concept of a middle-level health professional with a specified degree of independence, opportunity for significant advancement, and an aura of professionalism might be more appealing to these types of recruits than placing too great an emphasis on the dependency or assistant nature of the PA role.

It also must be remembered that each branch of the service trains and utilizes medics to meet its particular needs. While the Navy trains independent-duty medics to function aboard ship, the Air Force does not place medics on its planes; rather, the Air Force uses medical corpsmen predominately in hospitals and dispensaries where supervision is high. Consequently, the level and type of training received by Navy corpsmen is of a more intensive nature than that received by Air Force corpsmen.[55] These differences in prior education and experience received in the different services have been recognized by several of the PA programs. Of the 12 PA programs stating a preference for the ex-medic recruit, four specified that they preferred an independent-duty medic.

Each of the services in 1971 was beginning to develop its own in-service PA program.[56] The curriculum would be comparable to those offered in civilian PA programs; therefore, it was hoped that ". . . with a minimum of 'retreading' these military assistants could step into physicians' offices, clinics, and hospitals and begin work."[57] If, in fact, the civilian and military PA programs are to be developed using comparable guidelines, this would place still a third type of veteran source of health manpower at the disposal of the civilian sector. Short courses especially designed for military-trained PAs would have to be developed and an emphasis would need to be placed on developing equivalency and proficiency examinations to qualify for civilian certification as a PA.

By 1972, seven states (Arkansas, California, Colorado, Delaware, Florida, Iowa, and New York) had included specific provisions, within their PA-related legislation, to encourage the acceptance of equivalencies in lieu of part of a more formal educational preparation.[58] However, in at least one instance, this encouragement was not supported in the regulatory and administrative phase of the legislation. California's PA law, effective in September 1970, initially provided an example of a law which ". . . specifically allows and encourages. . . the use of equivalencies and proficiency testing to give full credit to trainees for previous education and experience."[59] However, these stated intentions of the law do not appear to have been completely carried out by the California Board of Medical Examiners who were charged with developing criteria and standards for this registration act. Specifically, the Board required a set period of clinical training for a PA wanting to work in California, adopted a detailed list of tasks a PA could perform, and required that an "approved" PA program should award academic credit equivalent to an associate degree.[60]

New York, on the other hand, has taken a very positive step toward providing active encouragement for veterans whose past training and experience might qualify them, with little or no further education, for a PA career. In order to encourage the qualified veteran to enter the new PA field (as well as other civilian health occupations), the New York legislature authorized establishment of a Veteran Health Manpower Center in the state.[61]

The discharged military medical corpsman has many very positive attributes which should promote his recruitment for, and success in, the PA role. Many of these attributes were mentioned by the program: relevant education, relevant experience, substantial supply, maturity, and a desire to pursue a full-time health career, as well as the fact that it is a predominantly male pool, which was felt to promote geographic stability, career commitment, and flexibility of working hours. However, there was at least one PA program in the 1970 survey which had found some reason to begin to question the too extensive recruitment of ex-medics as PAs:

> [There appear to be] certain disadvantages in accepting as surgeon's assistant trainees those who have had considerable experience as para-medicals in the military and have been in situations in which they were forced to make independent medical judgments without M. D. supervision. These individuals tend to be unduly self-confident, and must have considerable reeducation to. . . work in a dependent relationship to the surgeon.[62]

That the ex-medic should be recruited for the PA role is almost without question. Not only is the ex-medic being recruited by civilian PA programs but, as of 1971, major PA training efforts were under way in both the Defense Department and the Veterans Administration. In February 1971, the Civil Service Commission developed a job category and examinations for physician's assistants in which credit is given for experience as a medical corpsman.[61] Before too great an emphasis is placed on recruiting medical corpsmen, however, thoughtful consideration should be given to the resolution of some of the unique implications associated with such recruitment.

Other Recruitment Sources

At least seven of the programs in the 1970 national survey recruited high school graduates; this source was justified in one of two ways depending upon the nature of the PA training program. Those programs which defined the PA's role in very technical terms saw a need for a relatively short and technically-oriented training period; therefore, they felt that high school was a sufficient prerequisite. Other programs defined the PA as a product of at least four years of collegiate experience; they emphasized the need for maturity and of training a well-rounded individual; that is, one who could appreciate the social as well as the somatic aspects of medicine. Since the training program was itself so extensive, high school was considered a sufficient prerequisite.

There were approximately five programs that preferred two years of previous college experience. The rationale for this preference was more implicit than explicit in the available program materials; it appeared that the reason for two years of prior college was to provide some liberal arts background and, hopefully, some foundation in the basic physical and biological sciences. The one program that did require a baccalaureate degree (other than those requiring a B. S. N.) did so on the premise that college graduates were an untapped source for health careers; the program was designed to entice the "8-10, 000 young people who must make other career selections when they find that medical school admission is not available to them."[64] One might question the suitability or willingness of these recruits to assume a dependent supportive role in health care delivery having aspired to become independent medical practitioners. Encouragement of such recruits should be coupled with equal endorsement for a system of career advancements including the possibility of advanced placement in medical school at a later date.

There was one program in the 1970 survey that was unique; it was designed to recruit low-income indigenous people in a large urban area as well as recruiting ex-military corpsmen.[65] The rationale for this recruitment source was threefold: (1) people recruited from an area in need of health services are most aware of local medical problems; (2) they will probably prove most acceptable to the people they are to serve; and (3) they are most likely to remain in the immediate locale to practice after graduation. Thus, one program's solution to the recruitment problem reflected an attempt to correct the uneven distribution of medical services as well as the numerical shortage.

Several of the programs emphasized the importance of recruiting men into to health field. Arguments for the recruitment of men into the new job of PA were the availability of ex-military corpsmen who might more readily pursue a male-oriented profession, the fact that men appear to be more geographically stable once they are settled, and that men are less restricted by home and family responsibilities and therefore can more readily be available to the physician at all hours.[66] However, the preference of one sex over the other in the role of the physician's assistant depended greatly upon the type of PA being educated. If the PA was to be employed in orthopedics or in general primary care, often the male was preferred. If the PA was to be utilized in pediatrics, women (particularly older women with older children) were preferred. However, even those programs which explicitly acknowledged the desirability of recruiting males as PAs did not actively limit their selection to males.

ACCEPTANCE OR REJECTION FOR THE PA

In order to become an effective member of the health care delivery system in the United States, the PA must be accepted by existing health providers as well as by the consumer groups he will serve. The programs contacted in the author's 1970 national survey were requested to identify any variables which they had found to be important in promoting the acceptability of the PA by existing medical and other health professionals.

Important variables promoting acceptance of the PA by medical and other health professionals that were most often mentioned by the programs were: (1) the new health provider will be accepted if the graduates of the new programs do a demonstrably good job; that is, if they evidence maturity and intelligence and have a genuine concern for their patients; (2) the physician and other health professionals must be made aware of the need for these new types of health providers—and of the manner in which they will contribute to health care delivery; (3) to be accepted they must be well oriented to the concept of a team approach to health care; included in this orientation should be a willingness to recognize the physician as the leader of the team and thus be willing to play a dependent supporting role; and (4) they will be accepted if, in the area in which they work, there is a notable shortage of health workers; since the existing health providers will be overworked and will be glad to get additional assistance. Additional variables felt to be important in promoting the acceptability of the PA were: (1) allowance for sufficient flexibility in their job descriptions to promote maximum usage by their physician-employers; (2) if nurses were the PAs, they would be readily accepted since they are already legitimate health providers; and (3) if the major health professional organizations endorsed the PA's use, the rest of the health team would more readily accept this new provider.

Although in promoting the acceptance of a new professional one needs to be cognizant of, and promote, those variables found to be positively related to such acceptance, equal attention must obviously be afforded those factors which might augur the rejection of the PA. The variables most often mentioned by the programs as being associated with the potential rejection of the PA by existing health providers involved questions of professional jealousy and a failure to promote adequate understanding of the role to be played by the PA. With regard to the question of professional jealousy, some felt the PAs might be viewed as intruders into the nurses' territory while others felt that they would be viewed as intruders by many of the technicians involved in providing health care. Some felt that physicians were too independent and thus would not be willing to delegate a sufficient number of challenging tasks to make the PA's role a meaningful one. Others felt that the economic arrangements would give rise to professional conflicts; that is, nurses might feel that the PAs were overpaid compared to themselves while physicians might resent having to pay more for PAs than they now do for nursing assistants. With regard to the question of a possible lack of understanding of the PA's role, some felt that PAs would experience an identity crisis; that is, they would not have their own "bag of tricks" to claim as their area of expertise. In recognition of this potential problem, several programs emphasized the need to clearly define the roles, not only of the PA, but of all personnel on the health team; others felt that this problem would be greatly reduced by taking sufficient time when developing job descriptions for the PA to ensure that tasks assigned this new health provider would not compete with, or substitute for, the tasks normally delegated to other health and allied health professionals.

Several other factors which might lead to rejection of the PA were mentioned by the programs. They included: (1) lack of sufficient numbers of these new workers to make a substantial impact on the health manpower situation; (2) fear of added insurance liability, as well as related questions of legal status, which might prevent many physicians from utilizing the PA; and (3) continuance of obsolete medical practice acts which could prevent adequate legal latitude for the activities of the PA.

Acceptance by existing health professionals is essential to the viability of the PA concept. Equally important, however, is the general acceptability of the PA in the health care system, which would include acceptance by the public as well as by those in other health professions. Four factors were identified by many of the programs as being of the utmost importance in promoting the PA's general acceptability. The first was education of both the medical and lay community to the blatant need for increased health manpower so that the community would financially support and accept the use of the PA. The use of community meetings in order to interpret the new worker's role to the people and the use of the news media to make the public more aware of the need and the part the PA might play in its resolution were two of the ways which were suggested to achieve this education. Secondly, a substantial number of the programs stressed the need for existing professionals (for example, physicians and nurses) to promote the use of the PA through their professional organizations. Professional acceptance would lend the new PA an aura of legitimacy. The last two factors are closely related. One emphasized the importance of proper selection of candidates who are to become PAs, stressing the need for maturity, commitment, and intelligence. The second emphasized the need for demonstrated effectiveness; that is, the PA will be accepted only after he has proven his effectiveness over time. One program suggested that the way to measure the PA's effectiveness was not in terms of how much extra time the doctor has but rather if the people served are actually healthier at less cost.[67] The resolution of the medico-legal problems associated with the utilization of the PA, the availability of an increasing number and variety of needed health services not generally available at present (for example, home visits), and demonstrated national support for such programs were also mentioned as factors which could be important in promoting the general acceptability of the PA.

Acceptance of the Early Program Graduates

Since the success of an educational program is gauged by the success of its graduates, the programs in the author's 1970 national survey were asked to comment upon the types of positions obtained by their graduates and to share any knowledge they might have regarding their graduates' acceptability by physicians, other health professionals, and patients. In addition, they were asked to isolate what they felt were their graduates' most favorable and unfavorable characteristics.

None of the graduates of the programs were reported as having experienced any difficulty obtaining the employment for which they were trained. All of the programs stated that their graduates had been well accepted by physicians, other health workers, and patients. Depending upon the type of PA trained, PAs worked in hospitals, clinics, home health programs, and private physicians' offices. Since all of the programs were new and innovative, a number had attempted to follow up their graduates with varying degrees of rigor. One of the Pediatric Nurse Associate programs reported that they made it a practice to follow-up their graduates approximately eight to ten months after completion of the program. The most frequent favorable comment this program received from its graduates dealt with job satisfaction; the negative comment most often received involved the difficulty of role reorientation.[68] One graduate of a surgeon's assistant program experienced some difficulty in utilizing all of his acquired skills in the hospital portion of his physician-employer's practice; he was not allowed to carry out procedures which were to become part of the hospital's permanent record (for example, histories and physical examinations).[69] None of the other graduates of this program experienced any difficulties in their work experiences. The most positive characteristics seen in graduates of this program were their acceptance of a dependent role in relation to the surgeon-employer, while still maintaining considerable initiative in patient care within the limits of their skills and training, and their ability to establish good working relationships with other health professionals—particularly the nursing staff.

Several programs noted the enthusiasm which their graduates felt for their new jobs and, in turn, the high regard their employers and patients had for the competence they exhibited. However, at least two of the programs that were in late 1970 in the planning stage of development, admitted some anxiety with regard to the continued acceptance of the PA by his employer, fellow workers, and the patients. In particular, programs that train PAs (for example as anesthesia technologists) who have existing health professional counterparts (nurse anesthetists) appear to anticipate some discontent and possible role conflicts between the two groups.

Other Studies Look at Acceptance, Rejection, and Need for the PA

Many of the operative and planned PA programs in the author's 1970 national survey cited the results of surveys of need and surveys of potential acceptance of the PA that they had reviewed or had themselves conducted prior to initiating their own programs. Some of the programs had felt it sufficient to rely upon national or "other area" studies of need. They were satisfied that, based on others' findings, there was both a need and a market for their graduates. Other programs had felt it incumbent upon themselves to study specific needs in their own particular geographic or specialist areas or both.

Some of the studies cited were of national scope; others were statewide; still others were strictly of a local nature. Some studies focused on the opinions of one existing health provider group (for example, physicians) while others also looked at potential coprofessional, staff, or consumer acceptance—or all three. Some specified in substantial detail the type of new health professional about whom they were soliciting attitudes.[70] Others left the type unspecified; that is, they surveyed the need for a medical assistant of unspecified specialty, education, or role.[71]

It is informative to note the types of studies which provided much of the impetus and rationale for the development of this new health professional. Specifically, what studies were most often cited by the early PA programs as being influential, how did some programs approach the assessment of need in their areas for a PA-type of health worker, and finally, how successful were these attempts at anticipating both need and acceptability?

Several Influential Early Studies

The specialty area best represented among the existing and planned PA programs was that of pediatrics. Of 12 programs declaring a specialty in the pediatrics area, nine were NP programs and three were nonnurse PA programs. This early proliferation of training programs in the pediatric area was undoubtedly prompted by the early support and guidance given this field by two influential professional associations. In addition, many of the earliest studies of health care delivery took place in the pediatric setting. The impetus for these early studies was the acknowledged fact that pediatricians, the primary care physician for children, were in very short supply. In fact, one writer noted that the shortage of pediatricians would not be corrected by 1980 even if the majority of all medical school graduates were to enter pediatrics.[72] An early (1966) time-motion study of four pediatricians had revealed that much of their time was spent in providing well-child care, a substantial portion of which did not require their specialized knowledge.[73] Given the acknowledged shortage of physician manpower in this area, a reallocation of tasks among health professionals was needed.

An extensive national study of the membership of the American Academy of Pediatrics (AAP) revealed that, although a large proportion of pediatricians felt that greater delegation of specific patient care tasks to an appropriately trained allied health worker would result in more efficient child care, existing task delegation was primarily of a clerical or technical nature.[74] Physician productivity rate (the number of patients seen per office hour) was found to be directly related to the frequency of patient care task delegation in settings of all sizes; ". . . greater efficiency lies not in the size or financing of the setting, but in the setting's employment and utilization of nonmedical health manpower for patient caretaking."[75] Although many physicians acknowledged the benefits of such delegation and indicated their willingness to do so if ". . . capable trained personnel were available," the inadequote utilization of registered nurses already employed in pediatric office practice was apparent.[76]

One study found that only 21 percent of the average work day of pediatric office assistants (four of the six assistants in the study were RNs) was spent in direct patient care. More alarming perhaps was the finding that registered nurses ". . . trained for three years performed the same functions as medical assistants trained for six months."[77] When one examined the type of tasks considered to be patient care, one sees that, for many of the tasks, such a classification was indeed generous—examples of patient care tasks included taking and giving information, social conversation, escorting the patient to the examining room, measuring height and weight, taking temperatures, and preparing and giving medications and immunizations. The RNs in the study did no guidance or counseling and very little patient teaching.[78] Obviously, nursing's potential contribution to child care was not being realized.

Having established a need for task reallocation in the pediatric area, a number of studies attempted to analyze the specific tasks which were amenable to such realignment. Abraham Bergman et al. studied the tasks of four pediatricians and drew an activity profile of a pediatric practitioner in order to estimate the degree of congruence between training and actual job performance; in this manner, activities which could more appropriately be delegated to others were determined. It was found that

> several distinctive functions common to all four practices constituted the major portion of physician-patient contact time. Those common tasks do not appear to be complex nor are they major items emphasized in either undergraduate medical or residency training. Not all such tasks require the talents of a well-trained pediatrician; many could reasonably be delegated to auxiliary medical personnel.[79]

Specific areas which could be delegated to appropriately trained personnel included many aspects of preventive medicine and well-child care including child development, nutrition, and family and behavioral counseling, as well as the performance of a limited physical examination with an emphasis on differentiating between major and minor illness states.

Alfred Yankauer et al. found a significant discrepancy between those tasks pediatricians say they are willing to delegate and those tasks which are in fact delegated; for example, while 64 percent favored delegation to an assistant of the task of giving advice on feeding and development, only 22 percent presently delegated such functions.[80]

Robert A. Hoekelman isolated data on New York pediatricians from Yankauer's national study.[81] Again, the discrepancy between present delegation of both office-patient care tasks (for example, information on child care) and out-of-office-patient care tasks (for example, home visits for treatment of chronic illness) compared with opinions about proper delegation was striking. By comparing "actual delegation" with "would delegate," the tasks which might be reallocated to an appropriately trained assistant were visualized. With the exception of a "lack of available trained workers" and "insurance liability problems," less than 25 percent of New York's pediatricians considered any potential obstacles to the use of health assistants as "very serious."[82]

In addition to studies documenting the need for, and potential acceptability of, an assistant role in pediatrics, pediatric-oriented PA and NP programs received early and official endorsement and support from two major professional organizations: the American Nurses' Association (ANA) and the American Academy of Pediatrics (AAP).[83] This example of collaboration between medicine and nursing was initially more an exemplar of the strained relations between these two major professions.

In 1970, the AAP issued

> . . . unilaterally developed guidelines for the expanded training of nursing personnel to the ANA's Division of Maternal and Child Health Nursing for their endorsement. The requested endorsement was refused by the ANA pending input by organized nursing. Subsequent collaboration between the ANA and the AAP resulted in the January 1971 joint guidelines on short-term continuing education programs for pediatric nurse associates.[84]

The joint guidelines had an immediate effect on the developing pediatric programs with four of the 12 pediatric-oriented PA and NP programs in the author's survey citing this report as a basis for their job descriptions. This joint statement will undoubtedly provide further impetus for the orderly development of more pediatric PA and NP programs, provide for a substantial degree of uniformity between the new programs, and remain an example of the potential gains effective collaboration between medicine and nursing may provide.

Attitudes of Physicians

At least six of the 12 programs training pediatric PAs and NPs cited one of the previously mentioned national or "other area" studies as providing a sufficient rationale for the initiation of their programs and therefore did not conduct additional studies of need in their own area. Many of the other PA programs did not rely upon national or "other area" studies of need. Several did not conduct studies themselves because they (the educational institutions) had been approached by state medical associations[85] or state health departments[86] to begin a certain type of PA program in order to meet a need these practicing health professionals saw in the immediate geographic area.

Several state medical societies had participated in statewide surveys of their members. Separate studies conducted in Delaware, Wisconsin, and Kentucky all demonstrated a significant potential market for the skills of PAs by their respective members. A survey of members of the Medical Society of Delaware revealed that while only 58 percent of the respondents (no response rate was cited in the report) perceived a need for a PA, 75 percent stated they would use one in their practice if available.[87] The authors suggested that the discrepancy between "need" and "would use" might be explained by some physicians perceiving themselves as busier than their colleagues and thus requiring an assistant in their own practices even if generally the need for such help did not appear to be as great as their own.[88]

Based on a 32 percent response rate from all practicing physicians in Wisconsin, Robert Coye and Marc Hansen found that 61 percent felt some type of specially trained "doctor's assistant" was needed while 42 percent felt that, if such an assistant were available, they would use one in their practice.[89] Whether a physician would use a doctor's assistant, and what type of tasks he felt were appropriate to delegate to such an assistant, varied greatly by the type of specialty the physician practiced. Sugeons would use these new assistants more often than other specialists. It is particularly interesting to note that when suggested tasks to be delegated to an assistant were closely related to specialty skills of the responding physician, the response tended to be strongly negative; for example, while only 2 percent of practicing obstetricians in the Wisconsin study would delegate an uncomplicated delivery, 27 percent of pediatricians felt such delegation would be acceptable.[90] In general, the Wisconsin physicians viewed a doctor's assistant as one of two types: a surgical technician with some additional responsibilities for medical histories and routine postoperative care or as a medical assistant to assist the general practitioner, pediatrician, or internist in his office practice. In the latter capacity, the assistant's tasks would include taking histories, technical procedures, health supervision, and triage functions.

> It seems quite clear that neither of these types of doctor's assistants is thought of by physicians as being an independent health professional operating with a hierarchy of graded and prescribed responsibility. Physicians in the survey sample see assistants almost exclusively as technicians.[91]

Although the new assistants in Coye and Hansen's study are envisioned as technicians, many of the more complex but still very highly technical tasks (for example, aspects of the physical examination) are denied them in favor of delegating to them areas of medical care (for example, portions of the medical history) often considered by medical educators as being more professionally demanding than the former. Coye and Hansen suggest some interesting reasons for this apparent paradox: (1) the technical tasks contain an immediate element of risk to the patient; (2) the physician is action-oriented; the "laying on of hands" is a respected (and expected) aspect of medical practice; (3) there are economic considerations since a physician is paid for what he "does" to the patient; and (4) "routine" techniques can provide an important safety valve to the overworked physician.[92]

The Wisconsin survey did not attempt to differentiate between the responsibilities of the nurse and the new doctor's assistant. Most respondents apparently believed that if they had enough nurses there would be no need for new assistants. The authors suggested that an argument could be made for a nurse not being considered a doctor's assistant; because she has her own unique skill (nursing care), perhaps she should be considered his professional associate. Further, since many of the skills needed by an assistant do not require the use of nursing skills, a nursing education may be an uneconomical preparation for such an assistant role. Nursing has already developed a system of ". . . nursing assistants—practical nurses and nurses' aides. . . . Perhaps physicians should. . . follow the example set by nursing in establishing multiple levels of professional training and skill."[93]

A 10 percent representative sample of the membership of the Kentucky Medical Association was asked to react to the initiation of a proposed program to train Clinical Associates (CAs) at the University of Kentucky.[94] Based on a 71 percent usable response rate (187 total respondents) from the sample, Ralph Eichenberger et al. found that 63 percent felt that there was a need for some type of new health worker such as the CA. Of the 63 percent expressing a general need for such a worker, 68 percent felt a personal need for the CA in their own practices. The physicians felt that there would be a fairly high degree of acceptance of the CA by physicians and particularly by other staff members. Two years of college was seen as an adequate educational prerequisite for the new health worker followed by a 24-month training period comprising equal amounts of academic and preceptorship instruction. Regarding opinions on appropriate tasks to delegate to a CA, the majority of both general practitioners and specialists in the sample would allow this new health professional to take a history and carry out treatment procedures while a majority of general practitioners would also favor the CA performing a limited physical examination, making a preliminary diagnosis, and conducting a diagnostic work-up.

F.A. Riddick et al. found significant support for the potential use of an allied health worker by members of the American Society of Internal Medicine; examples of tasks suitable for delegation included home visits, nursing home visits, patient teaching, and parts of the history.[95] A separate study of primary care practitioners (internists, pediatricians, and general practitioners) in central Virginia indicated that 50 percent could use a highly trained office assistant. Some potential disadvantages cited by the physicians were possible disruption of the physician-patient relationship, loss of personal control of patient management, patient rejection of the new workers, and economic considerations; that is, the cost of employing a more highly trained assistant in light of what their activities would contribute to the income of the practice. The physicians overwhelmingly favored the use of a specially trained primary-care nurse in the role of assistant as opposed to the use of a trained PA with a medical corpsman background. Reasons for this choice appeared to be associated with the gender of most nurses, which it was felt would promote acceptability in caring for women and children, the perceived legal advantages of using an existing licensed professional, and the assertion that a man would demand a higher salary![96]

A study of physicians conducted by Barry Borland et al. also reported considerable support for the use of trained assistants.[97] Although decision-making power involving medical diagnosis and the prescription of a therapeutic regimen were not felt to be conducive to delegation, gathering diagnostic data and carrying out planned therapy were considered appropriate. Interestingly, a close relationship was found between a physician's specialty and favorable attitudes toward the delegation of tasks closely associated with his specialty; for example, obstetricians and gynecologists, more often than members of any other specialty group, identified routine prenatal checkups and uncomplicated or emergency deliveries as tasks appropriate for the PA.[98] These findings are contrary to those of Coye and Hansen cited above.

Attitudes of Health Professionals Other Than Physicians

Although many of the earliest PA studies focused on the attitudes of practicing physicians toward this new health professional, there were several early local studies of the potential acceptance of the PA by other health providers and by client groups. In an early study of the Clinical Associate in Kentucky, it was noted that, while patients, physicians, nurses, technical, and lay staff accepted him, medical students tended to regard the CA "as a lesser person. Most would not eat lunch with him, include him in their discussions of class activities, accept him as a laboratory partner, or share a patient with him in physical diagnosis. None ventured friendship with him."[99] However, it was found that, after the student CA completed training, his acceptance by the medical students increased.

A study conducted by Linda Breytspraak and Louis Pondy focused on both the PA's role-set acceptance (for example, acceptance by nurses, physicians, technicians, administrative personnel) and his self-acceptance in his new position.[100] The investigators found much diversity in the actual roles being fulfilled by each of eight early graduates of the Duke PA program; some fulfilled a "staff" role (for example, worked as a direct assistant to the physician), and others functioned in a "line" capacity, attached to an institutional sub-group with direct lines to the physician above and with some supervisory activities over technical personnel below. Generally both self-acceptance and role-set acceptance were high. However, the work situation that promoted one type of acceptance was not always the most conducive to promoting the second type of acceptance.

> Self-acceptance and satisfaction appeared to occur most frequently when the PA felt that he was carrying out unique functions distinct from those of other paramedical personnel and congruent with the ideals enunciated during the two year training period. . . role-set acceptance appeared to be high when the role-set members saw the Physician's Assistant as carrying out a set of functions visibly helping them in their own work.[101]

Role set members tended to be more conservative in their estimate of the potential scope of activities of the PA than the employing physicians who were not particularly concerned about limiting the PA's role.

Attitudes of the Consumer

An early study was conducted by Patricia Patterson et al. examining "parent reaction to the concept of PAs."[102] This study was based upon structured interviews of 145 mothers whose children received health care in one of the following settings: private offices, group plans, or public clinics. The researchers concluded that 75 percent of the mothers approved of the concept of a PA while 94 percent stated they would be willing to try the services of this new health care provider. Key determinants in promoting acceptance were the manner in which the concept was presented, prior experience with the use of some type of health provider other than the physician (most often a nurse), and prior trust in their pediatricians (for example, if he hired the PA, the latter would be competent). The positive advantages which the mothers anticipated from the use of such assistants were reduction in waiting time, having someone who would have the time to listen as well as to discuss health instructions in a more thorough and understandable manner, a possible reduction in costs, and a means of providing the pediatrician more time to take care of the sick children. Potential disadvantages envisioned by the mothers included the possibility of experiencing some discontinuity of health care if there were to be a rapid turnover of assistants, lack of communication between the pediatrician and his assistant regarding individual patients, and an increase in the impersonality of health service delivery.

An unpublished master's thesis studied the potential acceptability of ex-military corpsmen in the role of medical care technicians (a generalist type of PA) in rural communities.[103] Structured interviews were conducted with a sample of 25 residents in each of eight rural communities in Oklahoma who were experiencing a scarcity of sufficient medical manpower to meet their needs. The results showed that the residents would be willing to use the medical care technician for ". . . approximately 75 percent of their medical needs if he was located in their community and in contact by telephone to his supervising physician."[104] Distance from competent medical resources was found to be positively related to acceptance. In addition, both income and education were found to be positively associated with acceptance; however, the relationship with education was not statistically significant.* It was also found that the technician would be used slightly less often than the physician and that he would most often be used for routine and emergency health problems as opposed to those of intermediate severity. [An index of "severity of health conditions" was constructed, tested, and used by the researcher.]

Theodor Litman's study of the potential willingness of a random sample of rural residents in southern Minnesota and northern Iowa to use the services of ". . . specially trained former medical corpsmen to provide various medical services to themselves and their families under the supervision of a physician. . ." was conducted in mid-1970.[105] Based on an impressive 100 percent response rate (253 respondents), it was reported that 65.6 percent supported the notion of the PA in general. All but 14 of the respondents claimed to identify with a regular family physician whose endorsement of the PA would be very important in their acceptance of such a worker. Thirty-one percent stated they would have some concern over the adequacy of a

---

*It is interesting to note some findings of a study concerning the general utilization of physicians. Secondary analysis of data obtained from the National Health Interview Study found that better educated people tended to use physicians more often than the less well-educated; this was true even when controlling for income. However, the author cautioned that his finding should not be interpreted to imply that income is not an important policy variable in health care use; financial barriers are very relevant. See Murray Tucker, "Utilization and Price Analysis: Prospects for Avoiding Higher Program Costs in Health Care," American Journal of Public Health 209, no. 4 (July 1969): 529-533.

PA's training, experience, and ability, and 38 percent expressed a preference to be treated only by a physician if possible.[106]

Theodor Litman appeared to this author to be overly pessimistic in his reporting of services that the respondents were willing or unwilling to allow the PA to provide them. For example, Litman reports "greatest opposition" to the provision of prenatal and postnatal care as well as the performance of routine deliveries; Litman stressed that 26.4 percent of the sample were unwilling to allow the PA to render prenatal care, but equal emphasis could be placed on the finding that 47.8 percent were willing to accept this task. Although 43 percent were unwilling to allow routine deliveries by PAs, it is equally noteworthy that 30 percent expressed potential willingness to have this newcomer perform this highly emotion-riddled service. Finally, that 58.8 percent would allow the PA to provide postnatal care is certainly a very positive finding. Consequently, this author cannot share Litman's conclusion that, with regard to a PA's performing maternity-related services, ". . . there seems to be at least presumptive evidence that any attempt to utilize former medical corpsmen in this capacity is likely to face considerable public skepticism and resistance."[107] Other tasks that greater than 65 percent of the respondents would approve for the PA were routine physical examinations and history, simple emergency care including suturing lacerations, initial screening, and patient referral.[108]

Loring Conant et al. studied the anticipated acceptance of both PAs and new nursing roles by a random sample of households in two suburban communities in the Boston area. The communities were similar in terms of accessibility to health services but differed in socioeconomic characteristics; that is, one was classified as an upper middle class (median income $9, 043) community while the second was classified as a lower middle and working class (median income $6, 695) community. Based on an 81 percent response rate, it was concluded that ". . . members of the upper middle class community more readily accept the notion of their physicians' use of assistants and nurses."[109] The members of the former group were more willing than those of the latter to accept the PA's or nurse's performance of an initial evaluation of an acute illness, guidance regarding dietary problems, and suturing of a minor laceration. One particularly interesting finding was that the counseling role as well as the treatment of minor lacerations would apparently not be as well accepted as the tasks of history taking, laboratory testing, and preliminary evaluation of an acute illness. As previously noted, these former two tasks are to be included in the competence of both PAs and NPs; to be well accepted by patients, endorsement by the physician and general patient education would have to precede the delegation of these tasks.

All four of the studies cited above (Patterson, Fry, Litman, and Conant) were hypothetical; that is, they elicited consumer attitudes regarding their potential willingness to use the services of a PA if such services were to become available. Two other early studies of patient acceptability of the PA concept are also important to note since they elicited patient opinion after exposure to a practicing PA. Louis Pondy et al. interviewed 72 patients of four physicians employing PAs each of whom worked in one of four practice settings—public ophthalmology hospital clinic, private ophthalmology hospital practice, hospital-affiliated private allergy clinic, or a small community general practice clinic.[110] Of the 72 patients interviewed 57 had been treated by the PA and 15 had not. Patient education and income were found to be significantly related to the patients' acceptance of the PA. Specifically, a straight line linear relationship was noted between level of education and acceptance while a curvilinear relationship was noted between income levels and acceptance with the middle-income group ($5, 000-$8, 000) expressing highest acceptance.[111]

There is an apparent disparity between Conant's and Pondy's findings; Conant found the upper middle class group most accepting; it should be noted that Pondy defined his middle-income group at an income level roughly equivalent to that of Conant's lower middle working class community. Pondy found greatest acceptance in the middle-income group. However, both findings do appear to suggest that the least acceptance may be forthcoming from those groups at the lowest end of the income scale. Such findings will have important implications for the placement of the PA. While some have stressed the potential contribution the PA will make to providing care for the medically disadvantages (particularly for the urban and rural poor), others have been equally emphatic that in order to be most effective the PA must be introduced into the mainstream of health care. This is particularly important if charges of promoting two standards of health care are to be avoided. In this author's opinion, the findings of both of these studies provide at least presumptive evidence that the latter approach may prove most effective in both the short and long range; that is, with proper preparation by existing physicians, the middle and upper income groups may readily accept these newcomers; and once the PA is accepted into the mainstream of the U.S. health system, the lower income groups may find his use more acceptable.

Lewis Day et al. conducted an opinion survey of parents in the Denver area using the services of a pediatrician employing a pediatric nurse practitioner (PNP).[112] The services provided by the PNP were quite extensive, including conducting a thorough history and physical examination, screening tests, laboratory tests, home visits, health education, and anticipatory guidance. Ninety-four percent of the parents responding to the survey (68 of 94 families) expressed satisfaction with the joint care offered them by the pediatrician-PNP team while 57 percent felt the care provided was even better than that provided by the physician alone.[113] Disruption of adequate physician-patient communication is often cited as a possible disadvantage of introducing another professional into the health care relationship.

Interestingly, the Denver parents felt that they were able to maintain communication with the physician even though the time spent with the physician per visit was considerably less than under the previous practice arrangement.

Conducting surveys of the potential acceptability of a new type of health provider, prior to the new provider's actual introduction into the health setting, may be subject to criticism due to the hypothetical nature of the issue under study. Public opinion (including the opinions of existing health professionals as well as consumers) is always subject to change; attitudes only rarely accurately predict subsequent behavior. However, as Irwin Rosenstock has succinctly stated:

> The goal of understanding and predicting behavior should appropriately precede the goal of attempting to persuade people to modify their health practices, even though behavior can sometimes be changed in a planned way without a clear understanding of its original causes.[114]

It is exemplary of this philosophy that a number of hypothetical studies (studies that solicited opinions regarding the potential acceptability of a new health professional before he is actually introduced into the field) were undertaken. The author herself conducted a local case study of such a hypothetical nature, which is reported in Chapter 6. In addition to these hypothetical studies, a substantial amount of research evaluated the actual acceptability of some of the first graduates of the new PA and NP programs. Both types of studies have been shown to have contributed to the initial development, and consequent evolution, of the emerging PA concept.

LEGAL ISSUES CONFRONTING THE PA

The legal problems which may be associated with the use of the PA have already been mentioned as potential obstacles to the acceptance and effective utilization of this new health provider. In the author's 1970 national survey, the PA programs were asked to comment upon the means that each felt would be most effective in resolving the legal problems associated with the use of "medical judgment" by the PA. At least nine of the programs felt that the legal problems were getting more emphasis than they deserved; essentially, they felt that the physician-employer would be legally responsible for the PA since the PA would work under his supervision.

> Under the doctrine of respondeat superior, the physician is responsible for negligent actions of any person in his employ or under his supervision. The physician's liability for the

actions of the physician's assistant would be similar, therefore, to his current liability for the actions of his nurses and other office personnel.[115]

The Standard of Care Issue

Even though the physician may be responsible under the doctrine of respondeat superior, a central question involves the standard of care issue; that is, will the standard of care that is used as a guideline to determine if negligence has taken place be that of the physician or that of the PA? As queried in the Professional Liability Newsletter:

> So shall there be two legal standards by which quality of medical practice shall be judged when a patient has been injured? A first class standard for physicians and a second class standard for physician's assistants?[118]

The Newsletter suggested that, given the dual facts that the PA will be engaging in a limited practice of medicine and that he will be supervised by the physician, there may be a strong argument for applying the same standard to a PA as is applied to a physician. Only if a PA were performing a special task, unique to his training and not to that of the physician, would the application of a separate standard of care be likely to prove valid.[117] Thus, perhaps, the risk the physician-employer assumes in employing a PA is more akin to taking on a partner-physician rather than an office nurse or other type of office assistant?

The standard of care to which the PA and the NP will be held accountable is an issue which is likely to receive even greater attention in the future as the activities of both of these health professionals are subjected to judicial review. The 1968 ruling in the Brune v. Belinkoff case will undoubtedly have applicability. In this case

> . . . the court required an anesthesiologist practicing in a smaller city to meet the general standard of care applicable to all specialists in his field regardless of where they are located. The former rule was that a practitioner would be required to possess only the knowledge and skills of other practitioners of ordinary ability and skill in "similar localities with opportunities for no larger experience."[118]

The application of a general standard of care, void of locality bias, provides a strong case for the promotion of national program accreditation and national certification of the graduates of these new programs. It also suggests the necessity of providing continuing education for all health providers.

Legal Accommodation for the Nurse Practitioner

The majority of programs in the author's 1970 survey involved with educating nurses for an expanded role felt that, if anything had to be added to provide the legal framework for the nurse to function in the broader role, the only requirement was to expand the tasks now allowed by the various state nurse practice acts; in particular, such acts should be expanded to allow for the nurses' greater role in physical diagnosis and patient care management. An example of such legislation was introduced during 1971 to the New York State Legislature:

> . . . to revise the present New York State Nurse Practice Act, which will recognize nursing as an independent, primary and distinct health discipline. This will. . . provide a legal framework within which the nursing profession may continue to broaden its scope in relation to scientific and sociological changes.[119]

After passing both houses of the New York Legislature, a proposed amendment to the State's Nurse Practice Act was vetoed by the governor on the advice of the Hospital Association of New York State and the New York State Medical Society. Fortunately the bill was resubmitted in 1972 and was passed.[120]

Others have noted the ease with which nurses with expanded roles should find legal sanction for their activities. As expressed by Richard Bergen:

> Without any change in the Nursing Practice Act, in most instances, it is probable that delegation to nurses under physician supervision can be made of virtually any medical procedure that does not, on a scientifically determined basis, require the personal knowledge, skill, and judgment of a physician. This has already been accomplished with respect to nurse anesthetists without the benefits of any special statute. . .[121]

One should note the particular importance of one of Bergen's qualifying phrases: under certain conditions, one can delegate ". . . any medical procedure that does not, on a scientifically determined basis, require the personal knowledge, skill, and judgment of a physician." The implications of this phrase have been aptly noted by a number of PA programs. There can be no blanket acceptance of a level of medical judgment without critical analysis; each type of judgment must be critically analyzed so that a physician can defend his assignment of these tasks.[122] To provide a firm rational basis for the determination of medical tasks susceptible of delegation was the impetus for the thorough task analysis undertaken by J. S. Gravenstein et al. for the field of anesthesiology.[123] It was essentially the same reasoning which prompted the California Medical Association, through its Commission on Allied Health Professionals, to call meetings arranged by medical specialties, so that each particular group could establish a set of criteria related to its own needs and potential uses of a PA.[124] Undoubtedly, many of the findings of these meetings were useful to the California Board of Medical Examiners as they devised the regulations for the implementation of the 1970 California Registration Act for PAs.

Professional Liability

The issue of professional liability coverage was mentioned by several of the programs in the 1970 study as one which was of concern to many of the physicians in their area. Duke's PA program, after discussions with the major professional liability carriers and the Insurance Rating Board, were able to devise in 1970 at least a temporary solution to this problem. In essence, the board agreed to extending professional liability coverage to the hospital at no additional cost, to the supervising physician at a negligible rate increase, and to the university-trained PA at a rate approximately 50 percent of that charged the physician-employer.[125]

The 1971 case of Thompson v. Brent is important to the professional liability issue.[126] In that case, the court ruled that a medical assistant, without legal registration or license of her own, was negligent in her performance of a cast removal. The employer-physician, although not found negligent in his own conduct, was found to be liable as her employer for negligent conduct in her employment. As such, the physician's insurance carrier was ordered to cover the physician's responsibility for his employee's negligence.[127]

Frances Minno suggested a means of alleviating many unjustified malpractice fears associated with the employment of a PA by a physician.[128] On the basis of individual rulings by a state board of medical examiners, or similar regulatory body, rules would be promulgated governing the delegation of specific medical functions in specific circumstances; these tasks would then be defined as lying outside of medical practice. "The physician's malpractice insurance would then cover these permissible actions of his assistant if a patient is injured, because the assistant would not be acting within the physician's exclusive realm."[129]

Minno's suggested resolution was based on the premise that actions performed by a PA, or other medical assistant, would by definition not be medical practice. However, others might disagree with this position. In a policy statement in 1970, the AMA's Committee on

Nursing viewed the nonspecificity of both medical and nursing practice acts as strengths which allow for growth in the scope of both medical and nursing practice. Acknowledging the overlap of many functions between nursing and medicine, the committee asserted that ". . . the same act may be clearly the practice of medicine when performed by a physician and the practice of nursing when performed by a nurse."[130] One could argue that this apparent substitutive nature of many medical and nursing functions should be explicitly acknowledged in their respective legislation. If the PA is to be in fact a true assistant to the physician, he will be engaging in a limited practice of medicine, albeit under the supervision of a physician. Listing the activities that can be delegated to PAs does not make these tasks nonmedical ones; they are medical tasks that, on the basis of thorough analysis, are felt to also constitute a portion of the PA's recognized competence. Such lists, if developed, should be the product of a multidisciplinary board (composed of representatives of medicine, nursing, PA groups, allied health professionals, consumers) whose intent was to acknowledge the PAs', the NPs', and the allied health professionals' competencies in certain areas of medical practice as well as to recognize the unique skills of each group.

Toward a Legal Model for State Adoption

Two programs in the author's 1970 survey felt that a thorough examination, and possible reinterpretation, of the present medical practice and nursing practice acts of each state should be conducted to determine if any of the proposed activities of the PA would contravene these existing acts. Based on an interpretation of both of the appropriate statutes in North Carolina, the attorney general ruled that, as long as a PA was used in the proposed manner, Duke's PAs would not be in violation of the existing state legislation. Encouraged by the attorney general's opinion but realizing such an opinion has no legal significance in a court other than advisory, the Duke program felt that some specific legal sanction would be of value for the PA. Thus, in 1969, a conference was held at Duke University to consider appropriate means of accommodating the PA (as well as other new health personnel) into the legal framework of medical practice. It was hoped that out of these meetings would come a legislative proposal to be used as a model for states' adoption.

Although a nationally applicable state model could not be developed at that time, the Duke conference formulated and extensively discussed several potential approaches for providing the PA with some legal sanction for his activities:

> Five alternative courses of action were presented for consideration: (1) maintaining the status quo; (2) licensing

physician's assistants; (3) enacting a general statute authorizing supervised delegation by physicians; (4) special licensing of physicians to utilize physician's assistants; and (5) establishing a Committee on Health Manpower innovations to control the development and utilization of new personnel.[131]

At Duke, an emphasis was placed on the third and fourth options with the fifth to be instituted at a future date. Essentially, a general delegatory amendment to the state's medical practice act would authorize supervised delegations to a PA by a physician, both of whom had been approved by the appropriate state board of medical examiners. The state board, thus, would have the primary regulatory and administrative responsibility for the act, although it would be the responsibility of the physician to direct and supervise the PA's actual performance. An independent Committee on Health Manpower Innovations might possibly be convened at a later date to consider more long-range proposals.[132]

The use of a delegatory amendment was not a new approach. Several other states (for example, Arizona, Colorado, Kansas, and Oklahoma) had adopted general delegatory statutes prior to the introduction of the PA in order to allow the physician to legally delegate tasks to qualified assistants.[133] At least six of the programs in the 1970 survey mentioned a need for a delegatory amendment, similar to that proposed by Duke, to be added to their respective medical practice acts. In effect, such an amendment would allow the physician to delegate many medical functions to a PA working under his supervision, as a legal exemption under the act. Consequently, it would afford protection against charges of negligence per se that focus on technical violation of the licensure scheme rather than on instances of actual negligence.[134]

In late 1970, the Department of Community Health Sciences of Duke University submitted three alternative versions of their legislative proposal for PAs to the Committee on Legislation of the Medical Society of the State of North Carolina. After consideration, the selected proposal was transmitted to a study commission of the North Carolina Legislature, which, in turn, was to submit the proposal to the legislature in spring, 1971. The proposal, exception (14) to the definition of medical practice contained within the North Carolina Medical Practice Act, read as follows:

> (14) Any act, task, or function performed by an assistant to a physician licensed by the Board of Medical Examiners, provided that
> a) such assistant is approved by the Board as one qualified by training or experience to function as an assistant to a physician, and
> b) such act, task or function is performed at the direction

> and under the supervision of such physician, in accordance with rules and regulations promulgated by the Board.[135]

The proposal was designed as a permissive regulation act and not as a licensure act. It provided legal recognition as well as some legal protection for the dependent PA, but did not rigidly define their permissible scope of practice.[136] If a more formal specification of scope of practice was later found to be advisable, it would be the responsibility of the board, via a sub-committee, to develop additional guidelines.[137]

Essentially, by utilizing the Duke approach, approval and certification of a PA by a state's board of medical examiners would serve as a means of regulating quality. In addition, constant quality control would be afforded by the day-to-day supervision of the physician-employer. Most educational programs award a certificate to those who complete the prescribed training. A new graduate would contact a licensed physician with whom he wishes to work. The licensed physician, in turn, would make an application for the PA to the appropriate board of medical examiners, and if approved, the PA would become certified to work for that particular physician under his supervision. In effect, the PA would be certified under the license of his physician-employer. One PA program in the 1970 survey suggested the use of a slightly different mechanism; rather than the board of medical examiners passing on an application, a state governing body (composed of physicians, allied health educators, and public representatives) would be responsible for checking the physician's and the PA's qualifications.[138]

Duke's proposal did not require a strict employee relationship between the PA and the supervising physician. Consequently, it would be conceivable that a PA could receive his salary from a hospital as long as the PA was approved by the appropriate state board and was functioning under an approved physician's direction and supervision.[139] This possibility appears to be congruent with the previously cited position of the American Hospital Association.

The Licensure Issue

Most programs in the author's 1970 national survey agreed that licensure for the PA would prove too restrictive to the newly evolving PA role; however, some felt licensure would, and should, be instituted at a later date. Still others felt that licensure was an evil to be avoided—arguing that it would only perpetuate the "guild system" of medicine. One program felt very strongly that licensure was inappropriate for the PA since their independence as a profession ought to be limited. Supposedly, one of the avowed purposes for licensure is to protect the public against unqualified practitioners; however, one program emphasized that one-time licensure, as it exists today, does not provide a continuing monitor of quality as some would hope. Colorado is apparently the only state, thus far, which has enacted licensing legislation for the PA:

> The law provides for the [child health] associate to be examined and licensed by the Colorado Board of Medical Examiners to practice in association with physicians. . . who spend a significant portion of their time in pediatrics. . . . [Such associates] may prescribe certain drugs specified in the law; however, associates will not care for hospitalized patients or for those with serious or life-threatening illnesses.[140]

The Colorado law has included provisions to insure that the licensure of their child health associates will serve the function of quality control; that is, they recommend a renewal of the license at regular intervals with evidence of the maintenance of an acceptable level of competence, including proof that an adequate amount of post-graduate education is being maintained.

Martha D. Ballenger has aptly summarized many of the disadvantages of licensure, the traditional process whereby a governmental authority grants permission to qualified persons or institutions to engage in specified activities.[141] As presently administered, one time licensure does not provide the public with meaningful quality control of health professionals, nor has it kept pace with the enlarging competencies of existing health professionals working with advanced technology in more efficiency-oriented settings. Too often licensure has been a negative force defending the status quo and retarding legitimate innovation in the use of both existing and new types of health personnel. Recruitment, career mobility, optimal use of existing and new personnel have often been inhibited by a too strict application of formal educational criteria. Issues of professional jealousy become entangled with those of overlapping jurisdictions often leading to a less than rational resolution of the problem being evaluated.[142]

Recognizing the problems of existing licensure schemes, several professional and governmental organizations proposed a moratorium on licensure of any additional health occupations (including the PA) until a thorough reevaluation of licensure and alternative approaches to regulation could be conducted. In 1970, the American Medical Association (AMA), the American Public Health Association (APHA), and the American Hospital Association (AHA) were all advocates of this position.[143]

Institutional Licensure

Although in agreement with the current attitude against licensure, the majority of PA programs in the 1970 survey felt that some type of official recognition of the legitimacy of the PA role should exist. Two approaches toward regulating the PA's activities and accommodating this health provider into the existing health care system were proposed: institutional licensure and national certification of program graduates.

Two of the PA programs advocated the adoption of a type of "use license." Licensing of individual health professionals would be replaced by the licensing of institutions, clinics, or physicians' offices. "The prerequisites for such a license could insure the competency of the staff, such as board certification by the respective professions. Most medical training programs presently follow this type of system now; for example, internships and residency accreditation."[144] A similar approach would require the hospital or clinic to register qualified non-licensed health personnel to function under their supervision.

Nathan Hershey has been an early advocate of the institutional license.[145] Individual mandatory licensure of health professionals has often interfered with the most effective and efficient organization of services by health care institutions; too often legitimate questions of safety and competence are replaced by questions of legal technicalities alone. In order to promote the necessary flexibility to meet changing organizational needs as well as provide the public with meaningful quality control, Hershey suggests that:

> . . . individual licensing of practitioners might be legitimately replaced by investing health service institutions and agencies with the responsibility for regulating the provision of services, within bounds established by the state institutional licensing bodies.[146]

The state hospital licensing boards would develop appropriate job descriptions for hospital positions and establish qualifications for specific jobs in terms of both education and experience. Hershey maintains that it is the medical profession that has pioneered this approach in that, although legally a physician has an unlimited scope of practice, a physician's scope of practice within a hospital is circumscribed by his individual special education and experience.

The proponents of institutional licensure will have undoubtedly noted the support given their position by the recent (1965) Darling case decision handed down by the Illinois Supreme Court.[147] In essence, the decision held that the hospital was responsible for the quality of care afforded the patients within the institution by its physicians, nurses, interns, and other staff. "The modern hospital, in more and more jurisdictions is held legally and financially responsible for the quality of care rendered by all employed or affiliated health personnel, including physicians."[148] Thus, the concern the hospitals have expressed with regard to the use of the PA in the hospital seems justified; if the hospital is to be held responsible for the competency of the health providers practicing within the hospital, they have a right and responsibility to play a larger role in determining and overseeing the qualifications and utilization of these personnel.

National Certification for PAs

National certification of PA graduates, the second approach to legitimizing the PA role cited by the surveyed PA programs, has been endorsed and acted upon by the AMA and the National Board of Medical Examiners. Efforts toward developing a national certification examination for the PA were initiated in November 1971, after the AMA House of Delegates approved a document specifying educational standards for primary care PAs (Type A). Having developed standards for such programs, the logical next step was to develop a means of evaluating the graduates of approved programs. In addition, it was felt that a nationally validated examination could be offered to those with less orthodox educational backgrounds (for example, those with backgrounds as medical corpsmen) as a form of proficiency examination. Competence and not credentials were to be stressed.[149]

The methodology used in the development of the examination was exemplary. Under the direction of a special study committee of the National Board of Medical Examiners, identification was made of the health care tasks that a primary care PA should be capable of performing. These tasks were further differentiated on the basis of two criteria: frequency of anticipated performance in the practice of a primary care physician and how critical these tasks were felt to be to the provision of quality health care.[150] Having devised a set of priority-ordered health care tasks capable of being performed by a Type A primary care PA, an examination (with both academic and clinical emphases) was constructed and administered in November 1973.

To be eligible for the first national certification examination, a person was required to be a graduate or near-graduate of one of the approximately 60 approved primary care PA or NP programs—however, it is expected that the examination will be available to those with a less formal educational background in subsequent years.[151] The examination was designed only for assistants to primary care physicians; at a later date, consideration will be given to developing a similar examination for other types of PAs, particularly the specialist Type B.[152] Whether the states will accept the certificate awarded upon successful completion of the examination as one criterion for legally certifying PAs is still in question; however, representatives of both the National Board of Medical Examiners and the Federation of State Medical Boards of the United States feel that the examination will be welcomed by state medical boards as evidence of a PA's competency.[153]

By December 1971, 28 states had some type of law affecting physician's assistants. Lawrence F. Wolper provided an excellent discussion of some of the positive and negative aspects of both existing and proposed legislation in 17 states.[154] In essence, he concludes that the laws to date have been inadequate; they make the PA completely physician-dependent, do not encourage correction of the geographic or specialty maldistribution problems, do not promote sufficient job mobility, and finally, do not provide adequate direction to the regulatory boards; that is, the state medical boards have had to make decisions in too many "grey" areas which should have been more definitively resolved in the legislation.[155]

Whether one agrees or disagrees with Wolper's analysis, it is clear that, although there has been much discussion and activity on behalf of the PA and his legal status, many issues still remain to be resolved. Definitive resolution of these issues (many of which were the focus of the present legal review) will not only take further analysis but will ultimately be dependent on changes that will occur in the broader health delivery system. The present laws attempt to meet the present needs of a PA working in today's medical market; that is, a PA working in a one-to-one relationship with a physician engaged in specialty or general, private, solo or group practice. Tomorrow's PA may be faced with a completely new system; for example public or quasi-public regional health maintenance organizations (HMOs) overseeing a series of decentralized health care complexes. Legal analyses must anticipate these changes, where possible; at the very least, provisions for readily adapting the PA role to meet the needs of a changing system must be incorporated into any legislation that is to have a lasting effect.

CONCLUDING REMARKS

The emphasis in this chapter has been on the initial development of the PA concept. The concept has now become a reality. Each year more and more PAs enter the medical market. Many problems of their entry had been anticipated; others were only perceived after they were experienced by the first graduates of the programs; still others will undoubtedly emerge only after considerable time has elapsed. As any advocate of change is well aware, theory and practice never perfectly coincide; however, in this instance, considerable progress has been made in a mutual accommodation between the innovation and the system.

Although almost a decade has passed since the first formal PA program was begun, the PA concept is still in its infancy. Progress has been made toward more specifically defining the PA, his necessary educational and experiential preparation, and his role in various settings. Recruitment sources have been identified. Problems of acceptability have been examined from several perspectives, including that of the physician, other health professionals, the patient, and from that of the PA himself. Legal recognition of the PA is a reality in a majority of the states.

In Chapter 5, attention is again focused on many of these same issues. However, the emphasis is now on the evolutionary development of the PA concept. Specifically, an attempt was made to discern the longitudinal changes in the opinions and attitudes of the educators of the PA regarding important issues facing this health professional. Consequently, the 43 PA programs originally contacted in the author's 1970 national survey were recontacted in 1973. The results of this resurvey are presented in the following chapter.

NOTES

1. Charles L. Hudson, "Expansion of Medical Professional Services with Nonprofessional Personnel," Journal of the American Medical Association 176, no. 10 (June 1961): 95.
2. Ibid., p. 96.
3. Ibid.
4. Ibid.
5. Ibid.
6. Ibid., p. 97.
7. Eugene A. Stead, "Conserving Costly Talents: Providing Physicians' New Assistants," Journal of the American Medical Association 198, no. 10 (December 1966): 182.
8. D. Robert Howard and C. Emil Fasser, "Duke University's Physician's Assistant Program," Hospital Progress, February 1970, p. 49.
9. Letter from D. Robert Howard, M.D., Director, Physician's Assistant Program, Duke University Medical Center, Durham, North Carolina, January 11, 1971.
10. National Academy of Sciences, New Members of the Physician's Health Team: Physician's Assistants (Washington, D.C.: The Academy, 1970), pp. 1-14.
11. Ibid., pp. 4-7.
12. "The Physician's Assistant Programs," RN 33, no. 10 (October 1970): 43-46; Joseph Kadish and James W. Long, "The Training of Physician Assistants: Status and Issues," Journal of the American Medical Association 212, no. 6 (May 1970): 1049.
13. Joseph F. Donovan, "Increasing Medical Manpower" (Paper delivered at the meeting of the National Association of Blue Shield Plans, Chicago, Illinois, October 5-6, 1970), p. 10.
14. Joseph F. Donovan, "A Medical Corpsmen Project," California Medicine 111, no. 6 (December 1969): 490.

15. Legal-Medicine Foundation, "The Physician's Assistant is Authorized in California," Professional Liability Newsletter 2, no. 7 (September 1970): 1.

16. Donovan, op. cit., p. 11.

17. Lawrence F. Wolper, "The Legal Status of the Physician's Assistant," Hospital Progress, October 1972, pp. 46-47.

18. E. Harvey Estes, "The Duke Physician Assistant Program," Archives of Environmental Health 17 (November 1968): 690.

19. Henry K. Silver, "The Pediatric Nurse Practitioner and the Child Health Associate: New Types of Health Professionals" (Paper delivered at the meeting of the New York Academy of Sciences, New York, New York, March 28, 1969), p. 8.

20. Ralph W. Eichenberger et al., "The Clinical Associate: Rationale for Training a New Health Professional," Journal of the Kentucky Medical Association, September 1969, p. 678.

21. Henry Silver and Loretta Ford, "The Pediatric Nurse Practitioner at Colorado," American Journal of Nursing 67, no. 7 (July 1967): 1444.

22. Ibid.

23. E. Harvey Estes and D. Robert Howard, "The Physician's Assistant in the University Center," Annals of the New York Academy of Sciences 166 (December 1969): 903.

24. Ibid.

25. Ibid.

26. Letter from Margaret K. Kirklin, M. D., Director, Surgeon's Assistant Training Program, Department of Surgery, Medical Center, University of Alabama in Birmingham, Birmingham, Alabama, March 10, 1971.

27. "Physician's Assistant Program 1970-1971," Bulletin of Duke University 42, no. 6 B (March 1970): 10-11.

28. Martha D. Ballenger, "Legal Considerations: the Physician's Assistant," Hospitals: Journal of the American Hospital Association 45 (June 1971): 61.

29. C.Y. Shu, "The Physician's Assistant," Hospitals: Journal of the American Hospital Association 45 (June 1971): 16.

30. Ballenger, op. cit., p. 61.

31. Wolper, op. cit., p. 48.

32. D. Robert Howard, "Development of the Physician's Assistant Concept—Duke University," Appalachia Medicine, September 1970, p. 1.

33. Rashi Fein, The Doctor Shortage: An Economic Diagnosis (Washington, D.C.: The Brookings Institution, 1967), pp. 69-70.

34. Elliott A. Krause, The Sociology of Occupations (Boston: Little, Brown and Company, 1971), p. 118.

35. Fein, op. cit., p. 70.

36. Clifford L. Carlson and Gary T. Athelstan, "The Physician's Assistant: Versions and Diversions of a Promising Concept," Journal of the American Medical Association 214, no. 10 (December 1970): 1855.

37. Fein, op. cit., p. 22.

38. Carlson and Athelstan, op. cit., p. 1855.

39. Letter from George G. Mallinson, Dean and Chairman, Ad Hoc Committee on Physician's Assistants, The Graduate College, Western Michigan University, Kalamazoo, Michigan, January 29, 1971.

40. Patricia K. Patterson and Abraham B. Bergman, "Time-Motion Study of Six Pediatric Office Assistants," New England Journal of Medicine 281 (October 1969): 771-774.

41. J.S. Gravenstein, J.E. Steinhaus, and P.P. Volpitto, "Three-University Study of Manpower in Anesthesia," mimeographed (Department of Anesthesiology, Emory University, Atlanta, Georgia, 1970).

42. Letter from Donald J. Frank, M.D., Director, Pediatric Nurse Associate Program, Good Samaritan Hospital, Cincinnati, Ohio, January, 1971.

43. Letter from James H. Hensley, M.P.H., Director of Training, Marine Physician Assistant Program, U.S. Public Health Service Hospital, Staten Island, New York, March 16, 1971.

44. Fred L. Fry, "A Study of the Acceptability of the Former Military Independent Duty Medical Corpsman as a Medical Resource in Rural Communities." (Unpublished master's thesis, Oklahoma State University, May 1970), pp. 1-49. (Mimeographed.)

45. For example, see "Physician's Assistant Program 1970-1971," Bulletin of Duke University 42, no. 6 B (March 1970): 3.

46. Howard, op. cit., p. 1.

47. Hu C Myers, "The Physician's Assistant in the Community Hospital and in Office Practice," Annals of the New York Academy of Sciences 166 (December 1969): 911-913.

48. Robert W. Ewer et al., "The Clinical Associate: An Indiana Concept," Journal of the Indiana State Medical Association, March 1970, p. 235.

49. Hu C. Myers, "The Emerging Physician's Assistant," Maryland State Medical Journal 19 (September 1970): 69.

50. Robert A. Hoekelman, "The Pediatric Nurse Practitioner: An Analysis of Potential Training and Utilization in New York State," mimeographed (Department of Pediatrics, University of Rochester, Rochester, New York, January 1971).

51. Priscilla M. Andrews and Alfred Yankauer, "The Pediatric Nurse Practitioner at Work: Function, Role and Identity," mimeographed (Pediatric Nurse Practitioner Program, Bunker Hill Health Center, Charlestown, Massachusetts, December 1970), p. 1.

52. Nancy Hicks, "Returning Medics No Longer Spurned as Civilian Health Aides," The New York Times, December 13, 1970.

53. Editorial, Journal of the American Medical Association 213, no. 11 (September 1970): 1765.

54. Joan Goldstein, "Medical Corpsmen as a Source of Civilian Health Manpower for New Jersey," Medical Care 8, no. 3 (May-June 1970): 255.

55. Ibid.

56. John M. Blamphin, "Department of Defense may become a Major Supplier of Physician's Assistants for the Civilian Health Field," Medical World News, December 11, 1970, p. 39.

57. Ibid.

58. Wolper, op. cit., p. 48.

59. William J. Curran, "The California 'Physicians' Assistants' Law," New England Journal of Medicine 283, no. 23 (December 1970): 1275.

60. Alfred M. Sadler, Blair L. Sadler and Ann A. Bliss, The Physician's Assistant: Today and Tomorrow (New Haven: Yale University Press, 1971), pp. 101-102.

61. Wolper, op. cit., p. 48.

62. Letter from Margaret K. Kirklin, see note 26, March 10, 1971.

63. "Government Programs Promote Training and Use of Physicians' Assistants," American Family Physician 3, no. 5 (May 1971): 163.

64. Letter from John E. Steinhaus, M. D., Professor and Chairman, Department of Anesthesiology, Emory University School of Medicine, Atlanta, Georgia, January 12, 1971.

65. Letter from Mary N. Nettles, R. N., Instructor, Medical Services Associate Program, Brooklyn-Cumberland Medical Center, Brooklyn, New York, February 5, 1971.

66. Howard, op. cit., p. 1.

67. Richard A. Henry, "Professional Assistant and Associate in Medicine Program," mimeographed (Division of Community Health, Department of Medicine, University of Florida, Gainesville, Florida, September 1970), p. 2.

68. Letter from Donald J. Frank, see note 42, January, 1971.

69. Letter from Margaret K. Kirklin, see note 26, March 10, 1971.

70. Patricia K. Patterson, Abraham B. Bergman, and Ralph J. Wedgwood, "Parent Reaction to the Concept of Pediatric Assistants," Pediatrics 44, no. 1 (July 1969): 69-75.

71. Robert D. Coye and Marc H. Hansen, "The Doctor's Assistant," Journal of the American Medical Association 209, no. 4 (July 1969): 529-533.

72. Abraham B. Bergman, Jeffrey L. Probstfield, and Ralph J. Wedgwood, "Task Identification in Pediatric Practice," American Journal of Diseases of Children 118 (September 1969): 459.

73. Abraham B. Bergman, S. W. Dassel, and Ralph J. Wedgwood, "Time-Motion Study of Practicing Pediatricians," Pediatrics 38 (August 1966): 254-263.

74. Alfred Yankauer, John P. Connelly, and Jacob J. Feldman, "A Survey of Allied Health Worker Utilization in Pediatric Practice in Massachusetts and in the United States," Pediatrics 42, no. 5 (November 1968): 733.

75. ——"Physician Productivity in the Delivery of Ambulatory Care: Some Findings from a Survey of Pediatricians," Medical Care 8, no. 1 (January-February 1970): 45.

76. Alfred Yankauer, John P. Connelly, and Jacob J. Feldman, "Task Performance and Task Delegation in Pediatric Office Practice," American Journal of Public Health 59, no. 7 (July 1969): 1116.

77. Patterson and Bergman, op. cit., p. 771.

78. Ibid., pp. 773-774.

79. Bergman, Probstfield and Wedgwood, op. cit., p. 466.

80. Alfred Yankauer et al., "Pediatric Practices in the United States," Pediatrics 45 (February 1970): 521 (supplement), cited in Judith R. Lave, Lester B. Lave, and Thomas E. Morton, "The Physician's Assistant: Exploration of the Concept," Hospitals: Journal of the American Hospital Association 45 (June 1971): 45.

81. Hoekelman, op. cit., unnumbered.

82. Ibid.

83. American Nurses' Association and American Academy of Pediatrics, "Guidelines on Short-Term Continuing Education Programs for Pediatric Nurse Associates," mimeographed (Division of Maternal and Child Health Nursing, American Nurses' Association, New York, January 29, 1971).

84. Sadler, Sadler, and Bliss, op. cit., p. 77.

85. Letter from George G. Mallinson, see note 39, January 29, 1971.

86. Letter from Jean G. French, Department of Public Health, Director of Family Health Practitioner Program, School of Public Health, University of California, Berkeley, California, March 14, 1971.

87. John H. McGrath, Marjorie J. McKusick, and Bernadine Z. Paulshock, "Needs for Physicians' Assistants," Journal of the American Medical Association 214 (October 1970): 148.

88. Ibid., p. 147.

89. Coye and Hansen, op. cit., p. 532.

90. Ibid., p. 531.

91. Ibid., p. 532.

92. Ibid., pp. 532-533.

93. Ibid., p. 533.

94. Ralph W. Eichenberger et al., "Kentucky Physicians' Response to a New Health Professional," Journal of the Kentucky Medical Association, May 1970, pp. 303-310.

95. F.A. Riddick et al., "Use of Allied Health Professionals in Internists' Offices," Archives of Internal Medicine 127 (1971): 924-931, cited in Malcolm C. Todd and Donald F. Foy, "Current Status of the Physician's Assistant and Related Issues," Journal of the American Medical Association 220, no. 13 (June 1972): 1718.

96. Regina C. McCormack, Herbert M. Allen, and Eric L. Livers, "Family Doctors' Use of Office Assistants and Opinions Regarding Nurses in Primary Care," Southern Medical Journal 64, no. 4 (April 1971): 417.

97. Barry L. Borland, Franklin E. Williams, and David Taylor, "A Survey of Attitudes of Physicians on Proper Use of Physician's Assistants," Health Services Reports 87, no. 5 (May 1972): 467-472.

98. Ibid., p. 470.

99. Ewer et al., op. cit., p. 236.

100. Linda M. Breytspraak and Louis R. Pondy, "Sociological Evaluation of the Physician's Assistant's Role Relations," Group Practice, March 1969, pp. 32-33, 37-41.

101. Ibid., p. 40.

102. Patterson, Bergman, and Wedgwood, op. cit., pp. 69-75.

103. Fry, op. cit., pp. 1-49.

104. Ibid., p. 40.

105. Theodor J. Litman, "Public Perceptions of the Physician's Assistant—A Survey of the Attitudes and Opinions of Rural Iowa and Minnesota Residents," American Journal of Public Health, March 1972, p. 343.

106. Ibid., p. 345.

107. Ibid.

108. Ibid.

109. Loring Conant et al., "Anticipated Patient Acceptance of New Nursing Roles and Physicians' Assistants," American Journal of Diseases of Children 122 (September 1971): 203.

110. Louis R. Pondy et al., "A Study of Patient Acceptance of the Physician's Assistant," mimeographed (Department of Community Health Sciences, Duke University, Durham, North Carolina, February 1970), pp. 1-14.

111. Ibid., p. 7.

112. Lewis R. Day, Rosemarie Egli, and Henry K. Silver, "Acceptance of Pediatric Nurse Practitioners," American Journal of Diseases of Children 119 (March 1970): 204-208.

113. Ibid., p. 206.

114. Irwin M. Rosenstock, "Why People Use Health Services," The Milbank Memorial Fund Quarterly: Health Services Research I 44, no. 3, Part 2 (July 1966): 94.

115. "Physician's Assistant Program 1970-1971," Bulletin of Duke University 42, no. 6 B (March 1970): 6.

116. Legal-Medicine Foundation, "The Standard of Care Issue and the Physician's Assistant," Professional Liability Newsletter 2, no. 7 (September 1970): 2.

117. Ibid.

118. H. Creighton, "Changes in the Legal Aspects of Nursing," Hospital Progress, September 1971, p. 88.

119. Hoekelman, op. cit., unnumbered.

120. Sadler, Sadler, and Bliss, op. cit., p. 78.

121. Richard Bergen, "Irregular Assistants and Legal Risks," Journal of the American Medical Association 207, no. 6 (February 1969): 1231.

122. Letter from John E. Steinhaus, see note 64, January 12, 1971.

123. J.S. Gravenstein, J.E. Steinhaus, and P.P. Volpitto, "Analysis of Manpower in Anesthesiology," Anesthesiology 33, no. 3 (September 1970): 350-357.

124. Letter from Joseph F. Donovan, Executive Director, Santa Clara County Medical Society, San Jose, California, March 11, 1971.

125. Howard, op. cit., pp. 2-3.

126. William J. Curran, "Legal Responsibility for Actions of Physicians' Assistants," New England Journal of Medicine 286, no. 5 (February 1972): 254.

127. Ibid.

128. Franc P. F. Minno, "Unjustified Malpractice Fears are Preventing Use of Doctor's Assistants," Modern Hospital 116, no. 5 (June 1971): 71-72.

129. Ibid., p. 72.

130. American Medical Association's Committee on Nursing, "Medicine and Nursing in the 1970s: A Position Statement," Journal of the American Medical Association 213, no. 11 (September 1970): 1882.

131. "Physician's Assistant Program 1970-1971," Bulletin of Duke University 42, no. 6 B (March 1970): 7.

132. "Model Legislation Project for Physician's Assistants," mimeographed (Department of Community Health Sciences, Duke University, Durham, North Carolina, August 1972), p. 28.

133. Martha D. Ballenger and E. Harvey Estes, "Licensure or Responsible Delegation?" New England Journal of Medicine 284, no. 6 (February 1971): 331.

134. Ballenger, op. cit., p. 60.

135. "Model Legislation Project for Physician's Assistants," p. 38.

136. "Legislative Proposal for Physician's Assistants," mimeographed (Department of Community Health Sciences, Duke University, Durham, North Carolina, October 1970).

137. "Model Legislation Project for Physician's Assistants," p. 27.

138. Letter from Mary N. Nettles, see note 65, February 5, 1971.

139. "Model Legislation Project for Physician's Assistants," p. 36.

140. Henry K. Silver and James A. Hecker, "The Child Health Associate," Hospitals: Journal of the American Hospital Association 44 (October 1970): 47-48.

141. Ballenger and Estes, op. cit., p. 330; Ballenger, op. cit., p. 59.

142. Ballenger and Estes, op. cit., pp. 330-331.

143. Malcolm C. Todd and Donald F. Foy, "Current Status of the Physician's Assistant and Related Issues," Journal of the American Medical Association 220, no. 13 (June 1972): 1718-1719.

144. Letter from James H. Hensley, see note 43, March 16, 1971.

145. Nathan Hershey, "An Alternative to Mandatory Licensure of Health Professionals," Hospital Progress, March 1969, pp. 71-74.

146. Ibid., p. 73.

147. Anne R. Somers, Health Care in Transition: Directions for the Future (Chicago: Hospital Research and Educational Trust, 1971), pp. 27-28.

148. Ibid., p. 28.

149. Malcolm C. Todd, "National Certification of Physicians' Assistants by Uniform Examinations," Journal of the American Medical Association 222, no. 5 (October 1972): 563.

150. "A National Program for Certifying Physician's Assistants," The National Board Examiner 20, no. 1, reprinted in Physician's Associate 3, no. 1 (January 1973): 24.

151. "Physician Assistant Exam is Reached," Medical World News, May 11, 1973, p. 72.

152. Todd, op. cit., p. 566.

153. "Physician Assistant Exam in Reached," p. 72.

154. Wolper, op. cit., pp. 45-50, 67.

155. Ibid., pp. 49-50.

CHAPTER

5

CURRENT STATUS OF THE PA: RESULTS OF A NATIONAL RESURVEY OF EARLY PA PROGRAMS

In late 1973, the 43 operative and planned physician's assistant (PA) programs originally surveyed by the author in 1970 were again contacted regarding some of the major issues facing the PA. As previously noted, a usable response rate of 56 percent was obtained including 16 PA programs and eight nurse practitioner (NP) programs. The numbers of programs included in the restudy is somewhat small given the great proliferation of programs that has occurred between 1970 and 1973; however, since the programs included are some of the oldest ones and therefore pioneers in the area, their opinions and experiences over time should prove most valuable in guiding the future growth of the PA.

In this chapter, the results of the 1973 resurvey are summarized and briefly discussed. The data are organized and presented in a manner designed to reflect the uniqueness of the PA and NP programs, respectively.* Specific attention is given both to current opinions (late 1973) and to aggregate changes in PA and NP program positions (between 1970 and late 1973) regarding major issues; changes over time experienced by several individual programs are noted, when such is applicable.

DEVELOPMENT OF A DEFINITION AND APPROPRIATE JOB DESCRIPTION

The PA. The PA programs reportedly relied heavily upon the National Academy of Sciences' (NAS) definition of a Type A PA in defining their

---

*The PA program responses are separated from those of the NP programs; responses from each group are designated by the phrase "The PA" or "The NP" within each of the chapter sections.

health professional. (See Chapter 1 for the NAS definitions.) Specifically, 11 of the 16 PA programs cited this source as the primary basis for their definition of a PA. Naturally, many programs expanded upon the basic definition including characteristics that they felt were unique or particularly relevant to their specific programs. In essence, the PA was well trained in diagnostic and treatment procedures, able to assist the physician in all of his professional activities regardless of setting, was to provide direct patient services under the supervision of the physician who would be responsible for the assistant's actions, and finally, although proficient in technical procedures, the PA was to consider himself (and be considered by other health providers) as an educated professional capable of making certain decisions rather than merely carrying out direct orders.

The NAS guidelines also provided many of the PA programs with a foundation upon which to base the development of a job description for the PA. In addition, either supplementing or in lieu of reliance on the NAS guidelines, a substantial proportion of the programs employed several interesting individualized approaches to the task of constructing an appropriate job description. For example, several of the programs initially constructed a skeletal job description, which was more precisely defined only after extensive studies were conducted of how much, how fast, and how well the first students progressed through their programs. Others conducted their own analysis (or reviewed the results of previous studies in the relevant functional area) of the type of physicians with whom the PA would work; this analysis highlighted the tasks which were to be assumed by the PA; subsequently, the educational program focused on these tasks in developing the appropriate job description. Several programs reported that guidelines established by the American Medical Association's (AMA) Council on Medical Education in collaboration with the relevant professional association of potential physician-employers (e.g., American Academy of Orthopaedic Surgeons) were most useful to them in the early stages of their development. Still another approach reportedly used by a substantial proportion of the programs utilized the skills of an interdisciplinary committee (with academic, professional, and community representation), first, to develop broad categories of activities which a PA could be expected to assume, and second, to refine these broad categories with reference to the specialty orientation of the PA to be trained or the settings in which the individual would be expected to function, or both.

Although not reported as a major approach in the development of the job description, some of the 16 PA programs did consider the health needs of a particular target population and some did survey potential patients to determine what tasks performed by a PA would be acceptable to the target group and would most adequately meet their needs. Some programs followed both procedures. One program, which had initially relied extensively on the NAS definition coupled with an experiential approach to job description (that is, prepared their PA as a generalist and expected a more explicit job description to be derived by the PA and his employer once employment had commenced), stated that this approach had not fully met their needs. Given their experience with the program, they would have selected a more patient-oriented approach, examining the health needs of a target population and tailoring their job description to meet these needs.

The NP. Six of the eight NP programs in the 1973 resurvey had adopted at least some aspects of the definition and basic job description of a pediatric nurse associate/practitioner (PNA/PNP) developed by a joint committee of the American Nurses' Association (ANA) and the American Academy of Pediatrics (AAP) in their January 1971 "Guidelines on Short-Term Continuing Education Programs for Pediatric Nurse Associates."[1] The PNA/PNP is ". . . to assume a direct and responsible professional role in ambulatory child health care. The programs should build on previous nursing knowledge and skill and include some knowledge and skills that conventionally have been the province of the physician."[2] Experimentation in changing role relationships was to be encouraged. Specific tasks to be assumed by the PNA/PNP were securing and evaluating a health and developmental history, performing a basic physical examination, discriminating between normal and abnormal findings of the physical examination and developmental screening tests and making appropriate referrals, providing anticipatory guidance, recognizing and managing minor childhood conditions, carrying out immunizations, identification and referral to community health resources, making home visits when indicated, and engaging in collaborative decision-making with the physician and other health professionals.

Several PNP programs elaborated upon the basic ANA-AAP guidelines. The PNP was competent to give comprehensive well-child care, provide emergency care, be an "associate" of a physician, and be an intermediate health worker in the sense that she assumes some limited independent decision-making responsibilities that had previously been associated primarily with the physician; this expanded decision-making ability is based on her increased proficiency in the application of problem-solving techniques. While she assumes some medical responsibilities, she maintains the strengths of professional nursing practice—the teaching and counseling role, family care, and special concern for the psychosocial aspects of health and disease.

In addition to the joint guidelines, other approaches to developing appropriate job descriptions for PNPs were cited: (1) examination of the health needs of a particular target population and development of a job description to meet these needs; (2) use of an interdisciplinary advisory committee to develop broad categories of proposed activities, which were subsequently refined to reflect specialty and setting needs of the particular type of NP being educated; (3) incorporation of the results of task analyses of pediatricians into the educational program in order to provide NPs with the requisite skills; and (4) utilization of an experiential approach; after exposure to a generalist core curriculum, the individual NP, with her physician-employer, would develop a more explicit job description in the specific work setting.

One program educated two types of NPs: PNPs and Medical Nurse Associates (MNA). The MNA was to provide care for the chronically ill. Building on the nurses' present knowledge and experience, the MNA would function as a consulting member of a health care team, managing selected patients through follow-up office visits after the physician had diagnosed the organic disease and initiated treatment. This program envisioned each of its Nurse Associates

> . . . as an expander of health services rather than as a substitute for physicians' services which may be in short supply. There can be more effective utilization of physician time with the addition of the Nurse Associate but, equally important, there is possible fuller utilization of nursing personnel basic skills when additional skills are provided and when the role is redefined and expanded. [3]

The two remaining NP programs educated primary care NPs. The Family Nurse Practitioner (FNP) was an RN who extender her functional role to include practice modalities previously assumed only by physicians in the area of diagnosis and treatment of disease. The job description for this professional was based on a combination of two approaches: (1) a task analysis of the primary care physician indicated areas for needed competencies; and (2) initially utilizing a general skeletal job description, students were studied as they proceeded through the program in order to ascertain where needed changes should be made. Gradually, a more specific job description was developed. The second program had adopted the umbrella term "primary health care nurse practitioner" to refer to their four types of NPs including PNPs, School Nurse Practitioners, Maternal-Child NPs, and Adult Health Care Nurses. A primary health care nurse practitioner was defined as a licensed professional nurse providing direct primary, acute, or chronic care to individuals, families, and other groups in a variety of settings. While she is capable of independent nursing care decision-making, she functions as a member of a health care team and collaborates with other health professionals such as physicians and social workers regarding health care needs of her patients. She has considerable depth and competence in a particular field of practice, which enables her to assess the physical and psychosocial well-being of her particular patients, evaluate and interpret data to guide planned nursing interventions, and collaborate in decision-making and implementation of an approved therapeutic regime.

A NEW HEALTH PROFESSIONAL?

The PA. A majority of the PA programs in the survey classified their graduates as health professionals in contradistinction to allied health professionals. Several reasons were given for selecting such a classification: the PA is a clinician with limited but special responsibility for diagnosis and treatment; the PA is a health professional in his own right who is united to another professional, the physician; the PA is an integral part of the health care team who meets all the criteria of professionals and professionalism (for example, adoption of a code of ethics); the PA is trained to perform many tasks independently and with a competence level characteristic of a professional. The four programs that chose to classify their graduates as allied health professionals emphasized the group connotation of the term "allied" and the fact that the PA, although an associate of the physician, functioned under his supervision.

The NP. All of the NP programs classified their graduates as health professionals. Most felt simply that prior status as a registered nurse would automatically entitle the NP to such a classification. Several programs commented upon the need for each health professional to acknowledge and respect one another's competencies; the "mind-set" of every non-physician health provider being allied to the physician was not considered conducive to team delivery of health care nor the development of truly collaborative collegial relationships.

DEGREE OF SUPERVISION

The PA. The programs were asked to interpret a phrase often included in definitions of the PA, notably, that the PA is to "work with and under the supervision of a physician." Interestingly, the majority of the programs were in agreement with the following three components of a possible interpretation: (1) the apostrophe in physician's assistant is misplaced; it should be physicians' assistant; that is, the PA can be employed by a group of physicians or function under the auspices of a hospital's medical staff; (2) the PA can work in a setting physically removed from his employer as long as effective lines of communication are available at all times; and (3) it is sufficient that procedures performed by a PA be subject to "review as needed," for to require direct review of all procedures would unduly hamper the effectiveness of the new health provider. Only three PA programs felt that the PA must be employed by a single physician or that the physician-employer must be able to directly review all procedures performed by the PA, or that both of these requirements be met. One program noted that, although the PA could work for a physician engaged in group practice, the PA must always function under the supervision of his particular certifying physician and not under the supervision of any other member of the group. In keeping with this position, another program felt that, although a group or institution might pay the PA's salary, the PA would remain responsible to a single physician.

The NP. The NP programs were also asked to interpret what "working with and under the supervision of a physician" would imply for a NP. Seven of the eight NP programs agreed with the majority of PA programs; that is, the NP could be employed by a group of physicians or function under the auspices of a hospital's medical staff, could function in a work setting physically removed from her physician-employer, and would only be subject to "review as needed" of procedures considered to be within her realm of competence.

PRIMARY CARE PROVIDER OR SPECIALIST?

The PA. The pioneer PA programs have continued to emphasize the education of primary care PAs. Eleven of the 16 programs trained only PA generalists while three additional programs offered specialty options to be pursued after completion of a core generalist curriculum. Specialties offered were in surgery, pediatrics, radiology, pathology, obstetrics-gynecology, psychiatry, and anesthesiology.

The NP. The early NP programs have continued to emphasize the education of pediatric NPs. As previously noted, pediatricians are often classified as primary care practitioners; therefore, to call PNPs "specialists" may be inaccurate. Between 1970 and 1973, there has been greater attention paid to providing NPs for other types of primary care physicians. Whereas in 1970 seven of the eight respondents were educating only PNPs, by 1973 two of these programs had been expanded to provide education for additional types of primary care NPs, such as the Medical Nurse Associate. The eighth NP program educated a generalist—the Family Nurse Practitioner.

RECRUITMENT SOURCES

The PA. The programs were asked to indicate the recruitment source which they preferred for the role of PA. First choice preference was given by seven of the 16 programs to recruiting discharged independent-duty medics. In addition, four first choice ratings were given to both college graduates with a health-related major other than pre-med and to discharged medical corpsmen. The PA programs ranked potential recruitment sources on a scale from 1 to 4; that is, from first preference to fourth preference. Results of the rankings are presented in Table 5.1.

The reason most often cited for preferring one recruitment source to another was a perceived willingness and ability on the part of the selected type of recruit to assume a role of increasing responsibility requiring a substantial degree of independent judgment. This reason was very often given for selecting the independent-duty medic as the preferred recruit. The possession of a previously attained high level of general education and the willingness to train for, and function well within, a dependent occupation were clearly secondary reasons for any recruitment selection.

Although the majority of PA programs did not exhibit a change of preferred recruitment choices between late 1970 and late 1973, four programs now recruited primarily from different sources. Two programs, originally recruiting high school graduates or ex-medics, now preferred to recruit college graduates. The possession of a previously attained high level of general and health-related education was seen as an important factor in their particular recruitment preferences. One program, which had previously recruited registered nurses (RNs), now preferred ex-medics (independent-duty or general services), noting that these recruits would be willing and able to assume a role of increasing responsibility while still being willing to function in a dependent occupation. The fourth program had originally recruited predominately indigenous low-income workers in dead-end health jobs in order to simultaneously provide avenues of upward mobility for these workers and hopefully entice them to remain in the immediate geographic area, which was in need of many health services. In this instance, while still maintaining their previous objectives, this program now offered two different educational routes to the PA career—one led to the AA degree and one to the baccalaureate. While still recruiting indigenous workers, they now expressed some preference for the independent-duty medic or RN.

The NP. Quite naturally, all NP programs cited the RN as the logical recruit for the NP role; only three of the eight programs expressed any preference for the baccalaureate RN vis-a-vis the associate degree or diploma RN. Reasons given for recruiting RNs for the NP role were the availability of a substantial supply often currently ill-utilized, the willingness of RNs to assume a role of increasing responsibility requiring independent judgment, and finally, the possession by RNs of health education and experience to provide a firm foundation for advancement in the health field.

Only two of the NP programs were willing to consider appropriate recruitment sources for the PA career. These programs considered RNs (baccalaureate, associate, or diploma) to be appropriate recruits for

TABLE 5.1

Preferential Ranking of Recruitment Sources for the PA

Recruitment Sources	First Preference	Second Preference	Third Preference	Fourth Preference
Discharged independent-duty medical corpsman	7	4	0	1
Discharged medical corpsman	4	5	1	0
College graduate with health-related major other than pre-med.	4	2	2	0
RN with diploma or AA	3	2	1	1
RN with B. S. degree in nursing	3	1	2	1
College graduate with pre-med. not attending nor planning to attend medical school	3	0	4	0
High school graduate	2	1	0	2
College graduate with a non-health-related major	2	0	0	2
Practical nurse	2	0	0	0
Allied health professional (e. g., inhalation therapist)	1	1	3	4

Note: Numbers in the table represent the frequency of rank given each potential recruitment source by the 16 PA programs in the author's 1973 resurvey.

Source: Compiled by the author.

the PA role as well as ex-medics (independent-duty or general services), allied health paraprofessionals (for example, inhalation therapists), and college graduates with a health-related major other than pre-med. Reasons for preferring these recruitment choices for the PA role were similar to those given as a basis for recruiting RNs into NP careers.

THE NURSE AND THE PA

Recruitment of RNs as PAs

The PA. Recruitment of the registered nurse (RN) for the PA role continues to be a controversial subject; the positions of the major health professional associations on this issue have already been discussed in Chapter 1. Interestingly, nine of the 16 PA programs in the restudy favored such recruitment while five were specifically opposed to the use of the RN as a PA. The reason most often cited as a basis for recruiting RNs into PA programs was a belief that the goal of all health professionals is to provide the best health care possible to their patients; as a PA, the nurse would be able to broaden her skills and thus provide better care to her patients; whether she is called a nurse, a NP, or a PA should be irrelevant. Two other reasons for recruiting RNs were also often cited: (1) a RN becoming a PA is an instance of lateral career mobility at the very least and possibly an example of upward career mobility; such mobility should be encouraged in the health field since equivalent opportunities are often lacking in this area; and (2) the high degree of incongruity between nursing education and nursing practice has too often led to dissatisfaction with the nurses' role causing early retirement from active practice. Adoption of the PA role may keep many nurses active and interested in providing health care. (It should be noted that this is not the same as saying that the nurse-PA would be recruited from the ranks of inactive nurses.)

There was little agreement among the five PA programs who opposed the recruitment of RNs as to the primary reasons for their opposition. Cognizance of the present shortage of working RNs, which might be aggravated by such recruitment, was mentioned by two of the five PA programs as the most important reason for their position. Two other reasons were given secondary importance by two of the programs: (1) the belief that nurses who become PAs are changing their roles and thus are, in effect, leaving nursing; and (2) the belief that the appropriate way for a nurse to expand her role was to become a NP and thus build on prior nursing skills.

The NP. While five of the NP programs expressed serious opposition to the recruitment of RNs into PA programs, two favored such recruitment and one was undecided. The reasons given by these latter three NP programs for favoring the recruitment of RNs as PAs were similar to those felt to be important by the PA programs: (1) if a nurse-PA can provide better care to her patients with her new skills, what she is called (nurse, NP, or PA) should be irrelevant; and (2) noting incongruity between nursing education and practice, adopting the PA role may be a way of keeping many nurses active. Of the five NP programs opposing recruitment of RNs as PAs, two reasons were considered to be of primary importance to their positions: (1) NP programs build on nursing skills and understand the unique contribution nursing makes to patient care; if RNs wish to expand their role, they should enter NP programs and not be encouraged to become PAs; and (2) nurses who become PAs are not expanding their role; they are changing it; those who encourage nurses to become PAs are encouraging nurses to leave nursing. The use of professional nurses in the non-licensed PA career (potentially leading to legal difficulties) as well as the perceived dependence of the PA profession in contrast to the nursing one were both seen as minor although contributing factors to their opposition to such recruitment.

The RN, the NP, and the PA

Not only has controversy surrounded the recruitment of RNs into PA programs, but also some question has arisen as to whether the nursing role, after undergoing some formal or informal expansion (for example, the education of NPs or a restructuring of the traditional undergraduate nursing curriculum, respectively), would obviate any need for the further development of the PA. PA programs have a very definite interest in the promotion of the PA concept; consequently, they have very decided opinions on how the new PA role differs from, and complements, the role of the traditional RN and that of the new NP. NP programs should also have definite opinions on the role of the NP and how it relates to both the RN and the PA. Therefore, both the NP and PA programs were asked to note the essential differences they perceived between the traditional RN and the PA, between the traditional RN and the NP, and between the PA and the NP.

The PA. The PA programs perceived distinct differences between the traditional RN and the PA. The RN was considered to be primarily responsible for the provision of direct personal patient care as opposed to the PA who was primarily involved in diagnostic activities. The RN was trained to provide inpatient care, functioned predominately as an observer and recorder of facts, and carried out explicit treatment orders; this was in contradistinction to the PA who was trained essentially for outpatient care, was able to initiate treatment, and possessed procedural skills, such as laboratory testing, now often done by a vast array of allied health professionals. Different task competencies provided a basis for many of the distinctions made between the RN and the PA by the PA programs. The PA should be capable of performing such tasks as taking histories, physical examinations, suturing, casting, initial work-ups, some laboratory tests, and a multitude of diagnostic and therapeutic procedures—tasks that are not generally delegated to RNs. A final distinction between the RN and the PA was perceived to be one of independence; the PA was felt to possess a greater potential than the RN for making independent judgments and recommendations regarding subsequent testing, preliminary interpretation of diagnostic findings, and development of therapeutic regimes, albeit under the supervision of his physician-employer.

The NP. The NP programs, in turn, perceived several distinct differences between the RN and the PA. The RN was educated to appreciate the psychosocial aspects of health care, providing such care to patients and their families by her own efforts and by cooperating with other members of the health team. In contrast, the PA was a technician educated to perform specific diagnostic and treatment tasks (such as lumbar punctures and suturing). Adopting the "mind-set" of the physician, the PA was primarily concerned with disease states and not with health in the broadest sense. One program noted that in terms of preparation, the RN could do any tasks the PA is being trained to assume; in terms of implementation of these tasks, the PA can do only the less independent ones since his entire role is dependent on the physician.

The PA. Six of the 16 PA programs believed that the distinctions they had noted between the RN and the PA were essentially the same as those which they perceived to exist between the RN and the NP. While essentially in agreement with this position, the remaining PA programs preferred to delineate specific areas of competence that they felt were a part of the NP's role and not a responsibility of the RN. In essence, the NP role possessed a capacity for more initiative, more responsibility, and a higher level of independent functioning than the RN role. Greater procedural competencies were noted, such as conducting comprehensive physical examinations, laboratory tests, and initially identifying and appraising acute and chronic illnesses. PA programs saw the NP role as a melding of nursing and medical skills; however, the emphasis was placed on the expansion of medical skills it entailed and not upon a similar expansion of nursing competencies.

The NP. The essential differences noted between the RNs and NPs by the NP programs stressed differences in skill levels and in the degree of independent decision-making. In contrast to the NP, the RN has generally not been given the responsibility (or taught the requisite skills) to conduct complete physical examinations and health histories or function with a high degree of independence and confidence. The NP has more knowledge of the medical components of care and has more proficiency in providing total health assessments and primary care to her patients. It is her basic nursing knowledge upon which the NP builds, expanding both the nursing and medical components of her role. Thus, in addition to performing medical tasks, the NP should be competent to initiate and implement major nursing care assessments as well as engage in teaching, counseling, and anticipatory guidance activities.

The PA. Twelve of the 16 pioneer PA programs perceived no major differences between the PA and the NP. Minor differences were noted by several programs: (1) the NP would approach the patient with a different psychological set; she would maintain the mind-set of the nurse rather than fully adopting the mind-set of the physician; and (2) the NP is generally being trained in more limited specialties (such as pediatrics) than the PA and therefore may have a different impact on the system. One program noted that in their experience they had found NPs less able than PAs to follow appropriate leads and branchings when conducting a history and physical examination; this failure they felt would undoubtedly be corrected with appropriate changes in NP curricula. Another program attempted to explicitly differentiate between these two professions. In their view, the NP could prescribe and treat only on direct doctor's orders and could not establish even a preliminary medical diagnosis. In contrast, the PA could diagnose and treat within defined limits and care for many types of patients in a more comprehensive manner than the NP. Consequently, the PA was more physician-like while the NP was legally and philosophically tied to the nursing profession.

The NP. Only one NP program saw no essential differences between the NP and PA careers; both new roles differed from the RN in their assumption of diagnostic and treatment tasks previously performed by the physician. Another program was unwilling to differentiate in an abstract fashion between the two new professions; the basis for making valid distinctions between the two health providers must take into account the specific type of preparation of each individual professional as well as the setting in which he or she would function. In noting the major differences between the NP and the PA, the remaining NP programs stressed the technical aspects of the PA role and its overdependence on the physician. These qualities, they felt, were in contrast to an emphasis in the NP role on expanding nursing skills, increasing problem-solving capabilities, providing opportunities to make independent decisions based on nursing assessments of health problems, and requiring the assumption of responsibility and accountability for their own individual actions.

A Career Ladder for the Nurse?

The need for career ladders in the health field is an undisputed fact. Too often movement from one health profession into another is inhibited by the presence of strict licensure laws, the imposition of stringent formal educational requirements, the lack of proficiency and equivalency examinations to allow advanced placement, and the like. Although many health professions build on a common core of knowledge, there is little credit afforded a graduate of one type of program who chooses to pursue another similar health career. As previously noted, some PA programs do recruit RNs; however, there is no provision made for advanced placement due to the possession of a prior nursing education. Nonetheless, a RN entering a PA program is an example of career mobility; whether such mobility is to be considered upward, lateral, or downward career mobility or simply a complete career change has been debated. In the 1973 resurvey, the PA and NP programs were asked if they agreed or disagreed with an assertion that "the PA profession offers an upward career ladder for the nurse;" in addition, an explanation was sought for their positions.

The PA. Of the 16 PA program respondents, 11 agreed that the PA role offers an upward career ladder for the nurse, four disagreed, and one felt it would depend on the individual circumstances. There were several major reasons given for considering the PA profession an upward career ladder for the nurse: the RN as a PA would receive greater remuneration for her services, broaden her scope of responsibility, enjoy a greater degree of independent functioning, and receive an opportunity to play a role as a primary care practitioner with many medical competencies. Three of the programs cited present inadequacies in the nursing role as a basis for their opinion. Specifically, the programs noted the incongruity between nursing education and nursing practice leading to frustration, the gradual movement of nursing practice away from direct patient care, and the considerable available evidence of dissatisfaction in the nursing profession (for example, high job turnover). If the nurse is dissatisfied with her nursing profession due to these perceived inadequacies, then her movement into a nurse-PA role should be considered an instance of upward career mobility.

Four programs disagreed that the PA role offers upward career mobility for the nurse. Some felt that, although such movement would constitute lateral career mobility, one career could not be considered "higher" than the other. Another program felt strongly that the PA role was sufficiently different from that of the nurse so as to constitute a complete career change and should not be considered either an upward or lateral shift in career. Similarly, another program saw the NP or master clinician professions as providing the nurse with an "appropriate" career ladder, whereas movement of a nurse into a PA role would be a career change.

The NP. Six of the eight NP programs disagreed with the statement that "the PA career offers the nurse an upward career ladder." The reasons given for their positions were varied. One program commented that it was illogical to produce another group of "primary caretakers" when nursing, the largest segment of health manpower in the country, has never been allowed to fulfill the role it has defined for itself. In a similar fashion, two other programs believed that the PA was being trained to do what the RN should have been doing all along; the RN already has a role that is potentially equal to or greater than that being developed for the PA. The remaining three NP programs simply expressed general opposition to the RN becoming a PA; the PA role was "too technical" to be assumed by the nurse and should be considered a "dead-end career" because it would make her too dependent on the physician. The two NP programs that agree that the PA career might be considered an upward career ladder for the RN did so for only one reason: to date, the PA makes more money than the RN and, in our society, higher salary is often equated with higher status. Both programs felt that eventually salary differentials would be minimal between these two professions.

The RN in the Role of PA or NP

The RN, functioning in a new role as a PA or NP, is fulfilling a health provider role somewhat different from that which is presently assumed by most nurses. The PA and NP programs were asked two questions relating to this issue: (1) why they felt registered nurses were being asked to pursue careers as PAs and NPs; and (2) why they felt many RNs were apparently willing to undertake these new careers.

The PA. Two reasons were most often cited by the PA programs to explain the selection of many RNs to pursue careers as either PAs or NPs. One dealt with the potentially high degree of acceptability to be anticipated by the medical profession should the RN assume these new roles; traditionally, the RN and the physician have worked well together and thus the use of the RN as a PA or NP would receive strong medical support and acceptance. Secondly, RNs (including both active and inactive nurses) represent the largest pool of existing health workers; therefore, it is to be expected that innovative programs in health manpower would view nurses as likely candidates for their programs. A third reason, although given only secondary importance by the programs, was the potential offered by these new careers (if undertaken by nurses) to foster a more collaborative relationship between nursing and medicine. Interestingly, the potential for promoting public acceptance of the new PA and NP by recruiting nurses, the assumption that PAs and NPs would undoubtedly be recruited from the ranks of inactive nurses and thus not deplete the supply of active nursing practitioners, and the supposition that the use of licensed health professionals in new roles would lead to diminished legal problems were felt (by the PA program respondents) to be reasons of only marginal importance in the selection of RNs as potential candidates for PA or NP careers.

The NP. The existence of a very large pool of active and inactive nurses making them logical candidates for innovative health manpower programs was the reason most often given by the NP programs for the selection of RNs into the two new careers. Of only secondary importance was the medical support and general public acceptance which might be forthcoming if RNs were encouraged to assume these new roles. Similarly, the opportunity the new careers potentially afforded for promoting a more collaborative relationship between medicine and nursing should nurses assume these careers was given little importance. Significantly, no NP program felt that RNs recruited for either the NP or PA role would come primarily from the ranks of inactive nurses.

The PA. There was substantial agreement among the PA programs regarding the most important reasons for many RNs' apparent willingness to pursue both PA and NP careers. Nine of the 16 programs cited as the most important reason the potential the NP and PA roles afforded the RN to assume a greater degree of responsibility for patient care than she is often able to do in her present traditional nursing practice. Eight of the programs agreed that the second most important reason for the RN's willingness to enter these careers was the potential both professions held for advancement while simultaneously enabling her to continue to provide direct patient care. Too often promotions in traditional nursing practice entail movement away from personal patient care into administration or teaching. That the new career might offer the RN greater remuneration and that these careers might be perceived as sorely needed career ladders were not rated highly as reasons for the successful enticement of nurses into the new fields.

The NP. The NP programs were in almost complete agreement with the major reasons cited by the PA programs for many nurses' apparent willingness to pursue careers as PAs and NPs. The new careers would afford the RN more responsibility for patient care than she is presently given and would mean advancement (if she became a NP and not a PA) without removing her from direct patient care activities. Like the PA programs, the NP program respondents also saw greater remuneration and career ladder potential as minor factors in the RN's apparent willingness to become a PA or NP.

The PA. The PA programs were asked to classify, on the basis of their experience and general perception, both nurse-recruits for PA programs and nurse-recruits for NP programs. The programs were equally divided in classifying the type of nurse-recruits selecting PA programs; one half felt that nurses entering PA programs were generally disillusioned with nursing but currently active practicing nurses, while one half felt that such recruits were active nurses still interested in nursing but wanting to expand the skills they bring to their practice. Nine of the 11 PA programs who chose to classify nurse-recruits selecting NP programs saw such nurses as active professionals still interested in nursing but wanting to expand their practice skills. No PA program classified nurse-recruits for either PA or NP programs as disillusioned inactive or non-working nurses.

The NP. Only one NP program classified nurse-recruits for PA or NP programs as disillusioned with nursing, but currently active working nurses. The remaining programs saw nurse-recruits for either the NP or PA career as active nurses interested in nursing but wanting to broaden their skills as health care practitioners. In agreement with the PA programs, no NP program felt that NP or PA programs were recruiting disillusioned inactive nurses.

ACCEPTANCE AND REJECTION OF THE NEW HEALTH PROFESSIONALS

Reaction of Other Health Professionals

The PA. The PA programs were in virtual agreement concerning major factors necessary to successfully promote the acceptance of PAs and NPs by other health professionals. Of primary importance would be the ability of these new professionals to do a demonstrably good job as evidenced by intelligence, initiative, and genuine concern for their patients. The second most important factor would be the PAs' and NPs' willingness to work in geographic areas experiencing particularly severe health manpower shortages; for example, rural areas and urban ghettos. Two other factors were seen as important, though clearly secondary considerations, in promoting acceptance: (1) willingness of the PA and NP to work in specialty areas affected by severe health manpower shortages; and (2) promotion of sufficient flexibility in defining each new role and job description so as to encourage maximum usage by physician-employers making the new providers indispensable to the system. Commitment to a team approach to patient care, assigning tasks which do not substitute for, or compete with, tasks delegated to existing professionals, recruitment of nurses into the new roles, and endorsement by the major health professional associations were seen as negligible factors by the PA programs in promoting acceptance of PAs and NPs by other health professionals.

The emphasis placed in 1973 on the need for the PA and NP to visibly demonstrate their effectiveness to other health professionals was similar to that noted in the author's 1970 study. In addition, in the 1970 survey, there was perhaps more importance given to educating physicians and other professionals to the need for these new kinds of health providers as well as a felt necessity to clearly define the role of the new workers, particularly as they might infringe on areas which were at that time assumed by others on the health team. This seems a logical progression of concerns for those who wish to promote a new health provider; that is, in the initial stages concern is on promoting the idea and reassuring those who might be affected by the idea's introduction; later, when the concept is a reality, the concern of the advocates is to demonstrate the new worker's effectiveness in the system. In order to do so, the advocates must now assure that the system is willing to utilize the new professional in both an effective and efficient manner; consequently, the concern at that stage would be on educating physicians and others to the proper use of the new provider. As will be noted shortly, this is considered a major problem today by the promoters of the PA.

The NP. The NP programs were in general agreement with the PA respondents regarding both the two major and the two secondary factors that were felt to be important in promoting the acceptance of the PA and NP by other health professionals. In addition, the NP programs placed more emphasis on the important positive effects which could result from official endorsement of the NP and PA by the relevant professional organizations. This emphasis on the importance of objectively demonstrating the new professionals' effectiveness and on obtaining active professional support (both on a national and local scale) was similar to that expressed by the NP programs in 1970.

The PA. Issues of professional jealousy (for example, the PA and NP might be seen as "intruders into nursing's territory") and a failure to promote adequate understanding of the jobs the PA and NP are being educated to perform (from the perspective of both the new health professionals and that of the existing health providers) were both seen as potential impediments to successful acceptance by other health professionals. These two potentially damaging factors cited in the 1973 resurvey were substantially similar to an expressed concern in 1970 that the PA and NP roles must not compete with existing health professionals; the descriptions of the new roles were to be couched in terms that would show how they could be integrated with and complement the existing system.

Damaging factors of secondary importance, noted in 1973, were the continuance of obsolete state medical practice acts unduly hampering the effective growth and use of the PA and NP as well as a concern that, physicians being too independent, might be unwilling to delegate challenging tasks; the latter was particularly important in order to make the PA and NP roles meaningful ones, contributing importantly and visibly to patient care. Potential competition between employers (physicians) and employees (PAs or NPs), problems of economics, lack of availability of sufficient numbers of the new providers in a relatively short time to make an appreciable impact, and fear of added insurance liability were relegated to positions of marginal importance as factors which might impede the acceptance of the PA and NP by existing health professionals.

The NP. There were some differences in the importance attributed by the NP programs, as distinct from the PA programs, to factors potentially affecting the rejection of the PA or NP by existing health providers. While agreeing with the PA program respondents regarding the damaging effects of a failure to promote adequate understanding of the appropriate PA or NP role on the part of both the new providers and that of the existing workers, the NP programs felt that issues of professional jealousy would be of only secondary importance. Unlike the PA programs, the NP programs gave primary importance to the potentially damaging effects of obsolete state medical practice acts preventing needed growth in the scope of the NP role. Anticipation of added costs incurred in hiring and utilizing the PA or NP (for example, salary, added overhead, added insurance liability) as well as resentment by the physician or nurse coworkers of the higher salary commanded by these new professionals were rated as potentially important impediments. Although the opinions of NP programs in 1973 regarding potential rejection factors are similar to those expressed in the 1970 study, more emphasis is now being placed on economic impediments to the acceptance of the NP and PA and less importance is attributed to issues of professional jealousy.

Reaction of the General Public

The PA. Acceptance of the PA and NP by the general public is an issue of concern to those involved in the education of both of these professionals. The two factors felt to be of major importance by the PA programs in this regard were the quality of care offered the public by the PA or NP and the active support of and promotion of the new professional by other health providers (most importantly, the physician) to the public in general and to their patients in particular. An important secondary factor was the attention that should be given to educating the public to the need for innovative sources of health manpower and the ways in which these new providers would help meet this need. This factor had been given primary importance in 1970 when the PA and NP were just becoming visible in health delivery; having been introduced into many health care settings, there has been a change of emphasis from merely selling the concept to selling the actual provider and the quality of care he or she has to offer. Time as a factor in promoting public acceptance as well as the effect of adding a sufficient number of new and generally desired services (such as home visits) were felt to be moderately important in promoting public acceptance. Surprisingly, potential cost reductions to the patient resulting from the use of the new providers was considered to be of very little importance in promoting any significant amount of public endorsement.

The NP. The NP programs were again in agreement with the PA program respondents regarding the two factors of major importance in promoting public acceptance of the PA and NP. However, unlike the PA programs, the NP programs attached considerable importance to the NPs' and PAs' ability to make available services generally desired (for example, home visits) but often not provided due to a scarcity of qualified health professionals. Strong visible national support (in both a promotional and financial sense) was seen as a factor of some importance in promoting public acceptance, but a reduction in medical costs through the use of PAs and NPs was viewed as being of only marginal significance.

The PA. Three factors were given almost equal weight by the PA programs as being most potentially damaging to the successful promotion and acceptance of the PA and NP by the public. Fear of being subjected to "inferior care" or "second-class medicine," apprehension that the new health professional might interfere unduly with the desired primary physician-patient relationship, and finally, a desire on the part of patients to perceive their physician as a general family counselor readily accessible regardless of their state of health were all seen as potential problems affecting public acceptance. However, one program reported that they had surveyed potential public acceptance and felt strongly that none of these problems would have any serious negative effect on public acceptance.

The NP. The NP programs perceived only one serious problem potentially impeding public acceptance of the new professionals. Six of the eight NP respondents felt that the public might be apprehensive about the possibility of obtaining inferior care if they accepted the services of a PA or NP.

Acceptance and Rejection of Early Program Graduates

The previous question on acceptance-rejection factors affecting the PA and NP was designed to elicit knowledgeable opinions on these issues held by PA and NP programs. In an attempt to particularize these more abstract opinions, the respondents were asked to comment on their own graduates: the types of positions in which they had been placed; knowledge the programs had of the acceptability of their graduates in their practice settings by physicians, other health professionals, and patients; and finally, to note what appear to be their graduates' most positive and negative attributes. All NP programs had graduates functioning in NP roles; therefore, they were able to repond to the question. Five of the PA programs had not yet graduated their first class; one chose not to respond; therefore, only ten PA programs were able (or willing) to provide specific information on these issues as they applied to their graduates.

The PA. The variety of settings in which graduates of only ten PA programs had been placed was impressive. The graduates were employed with family practitioners in rural areas and with their urban counterparts, in group and solo private practices, in large urban hospitals and medical centers, in industrial health centers, in federal, state, and city prison systems, in public health departments, in satellite clinics, and as instructors in other PA programs. In general, the programs reported acceptance to be "good" to "excellent." However, only one program reported that they had determined the degree of acceptance by a formal evaluation: by the use of questionnaires and personal interviews with their graduates and their employers. One program noted that some of their graduates had experienced difficulties with hospital staffs accepting (and allowing) this necessary component of the PA role; another program's graduates had been criticized as being overtrained in diseases seen in tertiary care centers while being undertrained in diseases treated in primary outpatient care settings; another found that although their graduates had met with initial apprehension by their coworkers, after exposure to the new professional, the apprehension was displaced by enthusiastic acceptance.

Many positive attributes of the new graduates were cited. Examples of such attributes were a willingness to work in underserved areas, providing a special population (such as prisoners) with a high level of health care previously unobtainable, reliability and dependability as a primary care assistant, obtaining a high level of technological skill in a particularly exacting specialty (for example, anesthesiology), ability to function well as part of a health care team, providing care to more patients without an appreciable (or any) increase in cost of care to the patient, and exhibiting concern for the "whys" as well as the "hows" of health care delivery.

Negative attributes were also objectively noted. Examples of these negative attributes included an unwillingness to relocate from urban areas into underserved rural areas, too great a reliance on the physician-employer for their professional identity, overconfidence and willingness to perform tasks beyond their capabilities, too great a desire to relocate in order to receive greater remuneration, unwillingness to work "physician hours without physician pay," and lack of desire to engage in continuing education.

The NP. NP graduates were practicing successfully in a variety of settings. The graduates were employed in rural and urban areas, with private physicians (in solo and group practices), in hospitals, medical centers, and health maintenance organizations (particularly in their outpatient services), in public health departments, in satellite clinics and neighborhood health centers, in industry, in student health services (both in general school systems and in universities), in the military, in federally sponsored child health projects, and as instructors in NP programs. There were even NPs working as missionaries, in the Peace Corps, and on Indian Reservations.

All of the NP programs reported that their graduates were very well accepted by their employers, coworkers, and patients. At least four programs had conducted formal acceptability studies, the results of which had provided helpful information for their programs' subsequent development. One program studied acceptability of their graduates by the three major referents of the NP: physicians, nursing and allied health professionals, and patients. Acceptability by all three groups ranged from a high of 98 percent for patients (based on 1000 patient respondents) to a low of 75 percent for nurses and allied health professionals with the physicians expressing 90 percent acceptance.

Another program had recently evaluated 11 of their early PNP graduates.[4] While all graduates had been well received, some were better able than others to utilize their new skills in their practice settings. Several important factors affecting utilization had been noted: (1) in this instance, the most "ideal" utilization of PNP skills was reported by those nurses employed in a public health agency; (2) the availability and accessibility of medical back-up, in order to provide patients with on-the-spot referrals when necessary, was found to be an important variable for optimum utilization; this need not necessarily mean that both the NP and the physician must be located in the same office as long as provision for close contact was maintained; again, the "ideal" situation existed when both PNP and physician were employed by, or belonged to, the same health agency on a full time basis; (3) while a PNP in a pediatrician's office will probably generate more income than her own salary, funding may be a problem in many health agencies; this would have obvious effects on the adequate utilization and deployment of the PNP's skills; (4) the physician must want the PNP as a member of the health team—not just accept responsibility for her; and (5) in order to avoid charges of inequality of care based on ability to pay, it is essential that the difference in functions between the PNP and the physician be in terms of conditions treated and not in terms of type of patients seen.

A particularly thorough evaluation of their graduate nurse associates (PNA and MNA) had been completed by another of the programs in mid-1973. It consisted of two major parts: a patient encounter study and a role perception attitude survey.[5] In the patient encounter study, information was obtained from a nurse associate (NA) describing each patient visit she had made in a ten-day working period; this information was obtained after graduation, after 6 months of practice, and after one year of practice. The findings were based on a total of 2,751 encounters completed by PNA graduates. Private physician offices and ambulatory care centers provided the settings in which the majority of care was given; 93 percent of the patients were adolescents or younger; approximately one-third of the visits were for well child examinations, one-tenth for follow-up care, 18 percent for acute illness, and 16 percent for chronic illness. While the NAs took histories and performed physical examinations, screening tests, referrals, and so on, 24 percent of the total services performed related to health counseling and teaching of patients and their families.

The Role Perception Survey consisted of a mail questionnaire to 117 health professionals (physicians, nurse colleagues and supervisors, administrators, and the NAs themselves) functioning in the NAs' practice setting. With an 83 percent response rate (97 respondents), 80 percent reported that the NA was well accepted by patients; particularly high acceptance (80-86 percent) was noted in ambulatory care settings with somewhat less acceptability in private practice (63 percent). The NAs were themselves more critical of their acceptance level by patients—only 52 percent felt that patient acceptance was good. In addition, a number felt that their skills were not being adequately utilized in their practice setting. The degree of acceptance of the NA by other members of the health team was perceived differently by each of the respondent groups. For example, physicians perceived that 50 percent of physician colleagues accepted the NA well, and 74 percent of nurse colleagues felt that acceptance of the NA by other nurses was very good. While expressing some concern that the NA might miss some important medical problems or interfere with the primary physician-patient relationship, a substantial number of physicians saw a distinct advantage in being able to delegate many routine tasks to competent NAs. The nurses viewed the NA as a role model encouraging them to continue their own education and to assert greater independence in their own careers; the NA also served the nurses as a valuable resource person.

In addition to the positive attribtes of the NP graduates noted in the above study (for example, functioning as an accessible resource person), the other NP program respondents were enthusiastic about their graduates' abilities to perform successfully in the role for which they were trained. Their graduates were able and willing to make decisions, play the often uncomfortable role of change agent, and provide high quality care where it was previously unavailable (such as turning "shot clinics" into primary care centers). The NP graduates, in general, expressed high job satisfaction, were exceptionally thorough in the care they provided (for example, they were good data gatherers; were conscientious in developing and implementing therapeutic plans), and were able to offer patients comprehensive primary care, including a significant amount of counseling and patient education.

Graduates' negative attributes were also objectively commented upon by the NP programs. By far, the primary negative attribute of NP graduates appears to be their inability to fully cope with their role change; five of the eight NP programs saw this as the only important negative attribute of their graduates. For example, one program noted that too often their graduates were underutilized and yet were often unwilling to aggressively pursue better utilization. Still another program blamed the "traditional nursing orientation" as a reason for some of their graduates' reluctance to assert the full potential of their new role.

Current Major Problems Affecting Acceptance

The PA. The 16 PA programs were asked to comment on the single problem that they felt was the most important one to resolve successfully in order to effectively promote the use of the PA. Three problems were cited most frequently: (1) education of the physician to appreciate the unique competencies of these new professionals and to be willing to delegate appropriate tasks in order to maximize the PA's contribution to health care delivery; (2) promoting acceptance of the PA by other health professionals, particularly registered nurses; and (3) resolution of legal issues such as issues of national certification and passage of general delegatory statutes. Three other issues noted by several of the programs were also of interest. Two programs were concerned with the reimbursement issue, particularly as it might be affected by third-party payment policies. Another program saw a need to objectively evaluate, on a national scale, the contribution of the PA in order to visibly "prove their worth" to the system. Finally, one program had not yet found a method for selecting students who would make the best PAs in terms of attitude, aptitude, and long-range career commitment.

The NP. The majority of NP programs were in agreement regarding the single problem they felt most important to resolve in order to successfully promote the NP role—money. Adequate financing was needed both for the programs themselves and for their students (many of whom receive stipends either from the programs or, more often, from employers sponsoring them). Related to the funding problem was the issue of remuneration for their graduates; equitable salary levels need to be established for the new professionals vis-a-vis existing professionals (such as RNs) and other new health professionals (such as PAs). The effect of third-party payments on promoting the NP role was also mentioned. In addition, one program stressed the need to visibly demonstrate the NP's contribution by conducting an objective cost-effectiveness analysis of their value to health care delivery. Several other problems were also cited: (1) the need for a definitive statement from the ANA, the AMA, the AAP, and other professional associations endorsing the nurse and the NP as primary health care providers, albeit with back-up and consultation from medicine; (2) the need to educate physicians to utilize the skills of the NP more effectively; (3) the need to alter the archaic bureaucratic structure of many health agencies and institutions in order to allow NPs to function at their appropriate level; and (4) resolution of legal issues.

LEGAL ISSUES

Legal problems associated with the use of a PA or NP have been cited as potential obstacles to the acceptance and full utilization of these new health providers. Although there are many similarities in the types of legal problems which will be faced by both the PA and the NP, there are many unique aspects of the issues that are applicable to one or the other of these two professionals but not to both; for example, the NP already possesses a license as a nursing practitioner while the PA is a new career without prior licensure status. The PA and NP programs were each asked to consider separately the most likely and most potentially damaging legal problems facing PAs and NPs, respectively.

Legal Problems of the PA

The PA. There was significant disagreement among the PA programs regarding the most likely and most important legal problems facing either the PA or the NP. Six of the 16 PA programs felt that civil suits involving the doctrine of respondeat superior would prove most bothersome to PAs; that is, employers might not be willing to assume responsibility for negligent acts committed by their PA-employee particularly since "common custom and usage" might not yet be fully applicable to this new health provider. Five of the 16 programs saw civil suits involving the doctrine of negligence per se of primary importance to the PA; the doctrine might be applied to both the PA and his employer if injury resulted from an act committed in violation of an existing statute (for example, a state medical practice act) without regard to the actual skill or competence with which the care was given; such violation might be found to exist solely on the basis of delegation of tasks to, or performance of tasks by, unlicensed personnel. Only three of the 16 programs considered the possibility of criminal suits being brought against the PA for practicing medicine without a license and against his employer for aiding and abetting such practice to be a very likely legal problem.

The NP. Only five of the eight NP programs chose to respond to the question regarding the most likely legal problems facing the PA. Of the five respondents, three felt civil suits involving the doctrine of respondeat superior would be most troublesome, one saw civil suits invoking the doctrine of negligence per se as most important, and one felt that the PA might be subject to criminal suits for the illegal practice of medicine. (The significance of each of these potential problems was explained in the preceding PA section.)

Legal Problems of the NP

The PA. When asked to identify the most likely and potentially damaging legal problems impeding the use of NPs, five of the 16 PA programs cited the vagueness and ambiguity of nurse practice acts as presenting some possible legal problems for the NP. Present delegation of health tasks is often governed by "common custom and usage," which is very difficult to defend and document in a court of law. Even if such a defense were possible (and unerringly predictable) the NP has many new functions which are not traditionally considered to be part of the nurse's role and therefore could not adequately be defended in this manner. Coupling the vagueness and ambiguity of nurse practice acts and the fallibility of a "common custom and usage" defense, the NP may be legally vulnerable.

The remaining PA programs were equally divided in their opinions regarding likely legal problems to be encountered by the NP. Three felt criminal suits might prove to be a major problem. Two considered civil suits involving the doctrine of respondeat superior to be most likely; that is, employers might not be willing to assume responsibility for the expanded role of the NP, many of whose tasks have been traditionally assumed to be the sole province of medicine. Two of the PA programs thought that the NP might be most vulnerable to civil suits involving negligence per se. In this instance, the NP and her employer might be accused of violation of both a state's nurse practice act (that is, performing tasks which are beyond the scope of her nursing license and which are not officially recognized as being within the purview of a nurse's competence as established by "custom and usage") and the state's medical practice act (that is, performing or delegating "medical" tasks which are not officially exempted under the act) regardless of the skill or competence with which the care is given.

The NP. With seven of the eight NP programs responding to the question regarding legal problems of the NP, there was no agreement concerning the most likely or potentially damaging problems. Civil suits invoking the doctrine of respondeat superior as well as civil suits involving the doctrine of negligence per se were cited by two of the programs. Only one program felt legal problems would result primarily as a result of the ambiguity and vagueness of nurse practice acts; only one program considered criminal suits a likely or serious possibility. The remaining program stated that their NP program, one of the earliest, had experienced no legal difficulties and did not foresee any in the future; they had successfully amended their state's nurse practice act in 1973 so that NPs are now explicitly covered by the act and need only be licensed in the usual manner by the state board of nursing.

"A Small Degree of Independent Medical Judgment"

The PA. The previously cited 1970 National Academy of Sciences' (NAS) report on the PA suggested that the Type A physician's assistant could exercise "a small degree of independent medical judgment."[6] The PA programs were asked to interpret this phrase and to comment on legal implications which the use of such independent medical judgment might entail. Several PA programs felt that the phrase was "too timid" or, conversely, should be interpreted very broadly—the only restriction being in the stipulation of legal requirements for adequate supervision of the delegated activities.

Most interpretations of the phrase were expressed in terms of the types of tasks or situations in which the properly qualified and adequately supervised Type A PA could be expected to function with a degree of independence as expressed in the NAS definition. Such a PA might be capable of practicing in a satellite unit without the immediate presence of the physician; the PA could act independently in emergencies and in the provision of routine care; the PA can use independent judgment but only to the extent that the PA can integrate data and make decisions concerning subsequent non-life threatening tests to be ordered—any diagnostic or therapeutic decisions (except in emergency situations) must always remain with the physician. The latter qualifying clause was added by a number of the PA programs to the use of "independent medical judgment" by a Type A PA; given this qualification, several PA programs felt that an adequately trained and supervised PA could exercise some independent medical judgment with few legal ramifications. However, three programs felt that if a PA did exercise independent medical judgment (such as triage, treatment of minor illnesses, sprains, emergencies, instituting some diagnostic and treatment functions in specific circumstances), the PA would then be vulnerable to both civil and criminal suits. One program warned that the only way to insure adequate latitude for any degree of independent medical functioning by the PA was to pass appropriate legislation to permit PAs to legitimately act in full accordance with their capabilities and will full responsibility for their actions.

The NP. Only one NP program chose to interpret the meaning of a Type A physician's assistant's ability to exercise a small degree of independent medical judgment and to comment on the accompanying legal implications. Such a PA could diagnose, in specific circumstances, without a face-to-face consultation with a physician. The legal implications of such an act were those of responsibility and accountability; if a PA chose to exercise such judgment, he would have to assume legal accountability for his own actions as a separate health professional—not simply as the dependent employee of a physician.

Model Legislation for the PA

The PA. A 1972 Model Legislation Project, held in North Carolina, considered several alternatives for recognizing the legal status of PAs.[7] No final agreement was reached in support of a specific alternative or combination of alternatives; however, three proposals were felt to hold substantial promise of providing at least satisfactory interim measures.[8] Presented with a list of the initial six alternatives considered at the 1972 meeting, the PA programs were asked to select which of these alternatives they felt would be most effective at this time and which would provide the best basis for a long-range solution. Three of the programs felt that maintaining the status quo and relying on "custom and usage," along with the assurance that the PA would remain in a dependent relationship with his physician-employer, would be acceptable at this time; however, no program felt that such a solution held long-range promise. Interestingly, authorizing "general delegations" by a physician to his trained assistant, via a delegatory amendment to the state medical practice act, was viewed in a like manner; that is, it was seen as a strictly short-term measure. Licensure of the PA as well as the establishment of a multidisciplinary committee on health manpower innovations (to oversee the development of new types of health professionals during an initial period of experimentation) were given little support as either short- or long-term measures to recognize the legal status of the PA.

The majority of the 16 PA programs favored one of two measures to provide both legal protection in the short run and a firm foundation upon which to base a long-range solution. The first approach would be on licensing the users of PAs. Under this approach, the responsible licensing board would establish licensing criteria which physicians and institutions, desiring to hire an unlicensed PA, would have to meet before employing such personnel. This procedure would have to be followed each time a physician or institution wanted to hire a specific PA. A variation of this approach would allow the prospective employer to submit to the relevant licensing board(s) job descriptions for potential PA positions. Upon approval of these job descriptions, the board(s) would set qualifications necessary for an individual to assume these jobs. The user could then employ people who met these qualifications.

The second approach selected by many of the PA programs was a multifaceted one. After providing an exemption clause under a state medical practice act to allow delegation to a PA, both the employer and the PA to be employed would have to be reviewed by the state board of medical examiners. At a later date, a separate committee would be organized (under the state board of medical examiners) to devise definitions for the scope of permissible practice for PAs as well as defining what constitutes "proper" delegation by physicians. Finally, an independent multidisciplinary board or committee would be established to oversee the practice of all allied health professionals.

The NP. Five of the eight NP programs considered appropriate short- and long-term approaches to recognizing the legal status of the PA based on alternatives presented at the 1972 Model Legislation Project. Three selected licensure of users as the measure that would be most effective at this time. (This approach was explained in the preceding PA section.) One program also felt that this approach would provide the basis for a satisfactory long-range solution. The approach which was felt to provide a firm foundation for recognizing the legal status of the PA, on a long-term basis, was the multifaceted one mentioned by a substantial portion of the PA programs; that is, delegatory amendment to the medical practice act; review by the state board of medical examiners for both the PA and his employer; a committee to devise definitions of permissible practice for a PA; and finally, an independent board to oversee all allied health professionals.

The PA. When presented with the three proposals developed at the 1972 Model Legislation Project, the PA programs were divided in their support; approximately one-half favored the October Proposal[9] while the other one-half favored the Hershey Proposal.[10] The October Proposal consisted of four parts: (1) provision of an exemption clause to the medical practice act so that delegation of medical functions, supervised and directed by a physician licensed by a Board of Medical

Examiners, could be made by a physician to a physician's assistant provided the PA is approved by the Board of Medical Examiners in that state; (2) implicit in the Board's power of approval would be the power to deny or revoke such privilege when indicated; (3) the Board would develop guidelines to ensure that the appropriate degree of direction and supervision applicable to the particular situation and circumstances would govern the actions of both the PA and the physician or institution with whom he works; (4) the individual physician would have two functions: to evaluate his PA's capabilities and delegate accordingly and to provide "adequate direction" and supervision. This proposal would not require a strict employer-employee relationship between a physician and a physician's assistant; that is, the PA's salary might be paid by a hospital although his activities must be under the direction and supervision of a licensed physician. In addition, since the PA would be delegated tasks traditionally performed only by a physician, the PA's performance of these tasks must be up to the standard and quality of the physician's performance of these same tasks.

The Hershey Proposal was somewhat similar to the October Proposal in that it was also based on an exemption clause added to the state medical practice act. It did not refer specifically to physician's assistants; rather it allowed a licensed physician to designate functions, specified in a board approved job description, to a person who met the board approved qualifications for the job. As always, the licensed physician was to be responsible for directing and supervising the tasks performed by this person. It would be the responsibility of the physician to submit a detailed job description to the board. With or without the physician's assistance, the board would establish the necessary qualifications which the proposed employee must meet prior to employment. Although this proposal focused on the primary role of the physician-employer and his licensing board, a similar procedure could be established for the supervision of assistant positions in institutions.

The NP. The NP programs were divided in their support of any of the three proposals, presented at the 1972 Model Legislation Project, to provide recognition of the PA's legal status. There was, however, a slight tendency for the NP programs to select the Havighurst Proposal[11] in preference to either the October or Hershey Proposals. The Havighurst Proposal was very similar to the October Proposal in that it provided for an exemption clause to the medical practice act; however, it differs in two respects. It did not refer specifically to physician's assistants; rather, it allowed delegation, by and under the supervision of a physician, of tasks to "a person qualified by formal or informal training and experience to perform such tasks." Secondly, the board was not given prime responsibility for approving the prospective employee; primary reliance was placed on the employing physician or institution; the board would oversee the actions of physicians and their assistants by investigating complaints concerning improper delegations or the performance of these tasks by inadequately prepared assistants.

Legal Recognition for the NP

The PA. Recognition of the legal status of the NP in her new and expanded role has been the focus of some discussion. The PA programs were asked to consider approaches for legally accommodating the NP role in both the short run and on a long-range basis. The majority of PA programs felt that maintaining the status quo would provide adequate short-run legal protection for the NP. In this instance, the NP would continue to function under her present RN license with the assumption that current nurse practice acts, without revision, are sufficiently vague and allow adequate latitude to legally protect her in her new role. However, four of the 16 PA programs felt that, even in the short run, legal protection for the NP must involve an explicit expansion of the tasks allowed under state nurse practice acts, particularly in the areas of physical diagnosis and patient care management.

On a long-term basis, one of two approaches were most often selected to legally accommodate the NP: (1) explicit expansion of the nurse practice acts to recognize the NP role and its expanded competencies; or (2) requiring graduates of nationally accredited NP programs to secure a special license (via examination) providing legal recognition of the NPs' role in diagnosis, treatment, and some prescription activities. While several agreed with the need for an additional examination, some PA programs would substitute a certification exam in lieu of requiring a second licensure examination.

The NP. The majority of the NP programs (six of the eight respondents) favored one of two approaches for assuring adequate short-term recognition of the NPs' legal status: (1) maintaining the status quo assuming that, for the immediate future, the NP would be legally protected under her current nursing license; and (2) providing for an explicit recognition of the NP role in state nurse practice acts. This latter approach was also viewed as a satisfactory long-range solution by several of the programs. In fact, in 1973 two states (Colorado and Washington) had amended their state nurse practice acts to allow for explicit recognition of the NPs' expanded role. Issuance of a special license or official certification by the ANA and "an appropriate medical body" were two long-range approaches to legally recognizing the NP that were favorably mentioned by four of the eight NP programs.

Licensure for the PA?

Licensure for the PA has been the focal point of continuing debate. As noted in Chapter 4, several professional and governmental organizations urged a two-year moratorium (beginning in 1971) on the licensure of any new health providers in order to allow time to evaluate the advantages and disadvantages of licensure. The PA and NP programs were both asked to specify the major advantages (if any) and disadvantages (if any) of encouraging licensure for the PA.

The PA. Nine of the 16 PA programs saw no advantages to licensing the PA. Of the five programs citing advantages to licensure, four felt that licensure would provide some legal protection for the PA and his employer from charges of civil and criminal liability, and five viewed licensure as a means of promoting the geographic mobility (assuming the existence of licensure reciprocity among the states) of the PA. Protection of the public by insuring minimum qualifications of the practitioner and enhancing the status of the new professional were both seen as advantages of somewhat lesser importance.

The NP. Four of the eight NP program respondents felt that there were no advantages to licensing the PA. The remaining four programs perceived advantages only of a defensive nature; that is, licensing the PA would protect the PA and his employer from charges of civil and criminal liability and protect the public by insuring that the PA would possess at least minimum qualifications to practice within his officially delineated areas of expertise.

The PA. When asked to cite disadvantages (if any) of licensure for the PA, only two PA programs foresaw no disadvantages to such licensure. Nine of the 16 programs thought that licensure would be too restrictive for the new PA role; licensure would sharply limit the natural evolution of the new career and thus diminish the potential contribution of an approach designed to at least partially alleviate the health manpower shortage. Seven felt the major disadvantage of licensure would be in the fragmentation of health care delivery that it would encourage by reinforcing sharp (and often functionally irrelevant) boundaries between the diverse health professions. A disadvantage of secondary importance was seen as the potential impossibility of deriving an adequate license for the PA; the functional sphere of the PA would be determined by the setting in which he works (for example, hospital, office, clinic), his employer (for example, general practitioner, specialty physician, institution), and his formal educational or informal experiential qualifications or both. Conceivably, there could (and should) be as many types of PAs as there are possible combinations of these variables. That licensure might be perpetuating the "guild system" of medicine, that it could potentially restrict occupational mobility by setting rigid formal educational requirements for entry, and that it might be considered inappropriate for the dependent PA profession were all relegated to positions of marginal consideration.

The NP. Only two of the NP programs perceived no disadvantages to licensing the PA. The remaining NP programs were in general agreement with the PA programs. The two major disadvantages to PA licensure cited by these NP programs were: (1) licensure might prove too restrictive for the newly evolving PA role; and (2) licensure of still another health professional might encourage undesirable fragmentation of health care delivery. Interestingly, only one NP program felt that licensure was inappropriate for the dependent PA whose independence as a separate health professional ought to be controlled.

COST FACTORS

Effect on Cost to the Patient

The PA. The cost of health care has risen rapidly in the last decade. If, and in what manner, the use of PAs and NPs affect these costs may determine the ultimate impact each of these new health professionals will make on our health care system. Ten of the 16 PA programs felt that the use of the PA and the NP will have no appreciable effect on the cost of medical care to the patient. Although the use of the PA and the NP will be associated with an increased quality of care being offered to an increased number of patients, the physician will have greater overhead, including the addition of another salary to pay, extra facilities in which to provide care for more patients, and additional time spent in supervision. Consequently, the new income generated by these new professionals will be used to offset these additional expenses and the end result will be no appreciable effect on ultimate costs to the individual patient. One program noted that, although overall costs to the patient may decline, the individual patient will not see the difference reflected in lower prices.

Two programs cited the pricing system employed in medical care (fee-for-service-rendered) as the reason why the use of the NP and PA will have no appreciable effect on patient medical costs; that is, patient charges are based on the delivery of a specific service to the patient; the service will continue to be delivered under the physician's supervision regardless of who actually delivers the care. Another program believed that this situation might be altered by introducing the PA and NP into health maintenance organizations (HMOs). Use of these new professionals in HMOs might allow for the provision of less expensive services while still providing more comprehensive services to more patients. Finally, several programs commented that only after sufficient numbers of PAs and NPs are utilized in health delivery will their use force an appreciable decrease in prices.

While the majority of PA programs felt that the PA and NP would have no appreciable effect on patient costs, the remaining five programs were divided in their opinion. Three PA programs foresaw a downward influence on medical care costs to the patient resulting from the use of these two providers. PAs and NPs would be doing many of the tasks presently assumed by the physician; the physician would therefore be able to make more efficient use of his time. The cost of the physician's time contributes significantly to the high cost of outpatient care; thus, the lower employment costs of PAs and NPs (because of less training) should result in lower costs to the patient. Whether reductions in the cost of providing many services by using less expensive personnel would actually be passed on to the patient in the form of lower fees was, however, questioned by at least one of the PA programs.

One PA program saw the PA and the NP as a means to contain the cost of medical care. By increasing the number of patients a physician could care for, his gross income would increase without any appreciable increase in overhead; therefore, the physician could increase his income without increasing the price of health services to his patients. The remaining PA program felt that although the patients would receive more attention and better care as the result of introducing the PA and NP, salary and overhead expenses would probably be passed on directly to the consumer of these better services resulting in increases in patient costs.

The NP. Six of the eight NP programs felt that the use of the PA and NP would ultimately decrease the cost of medical care to the patient. No NP program saw the use of these health professionals resulting in an increase in costs, while two felt there would be no appreciable effect on patient costs. A decrease in costs to the patient would result from either of two factors. Physician services are very costly to the patient; many of these services can be provided by NPs and PAs whose salaries are considerably lower than those of physicians; the result should be more care to more people at less cost, since much of the care will be provided by the less costly professionals. Physician services could then be more readily available for those cases where their special medical expertise is required and thus result in the more efficient utilization of a "scarce and costly commodity." Secondly, a decrease in cost might result from the patients' more efficient use of the system; that is, good health care (including a substantial amount of patient education) would be available to more people thus encouraging them to seek "early and appropriate" treatment; this should be reflected in less use of the system for "costly crisis care" resulting in better utilization of services—and more importantly, better health for more people.

The setting in which the PA and NP services would be employed was seen as an important variable affecting cost by several of the NP programs. The skills of NPs and PAs working in HMO-type organizations would be most efficiently deployed to provide care formerly provided only by highly paid physicians. In other settings (for example, private offices and public health departments), although the PA and NP would expand the availability of services, their use might not have the same effect on patient costs. In this latter instance, although services might increase in both quantity and quality, there would be no appreciable effect on cost to the patient.

Salary Potential

The effect the PA and NP will have on the cost of medical care to the patient is only one of the relevant cost issues involved in the development of these new health professionals. Other issues of importance are approximate annual salaries of graduates, training costs, and the role of third-party payments.*

How the salaries of the NP and PA will be paid was not explicitly discussed by the program respondents. To date, most of these health providers have been paid on a salaried basis by the physician- or institution-employer. Patient charges to cover the cost of these salaries have generally been on a fee-for-service basis, charging the patient

---

*Productivity also has implications for the economic viability of the PA and NP. Task analysis has focused attention on the time physicians spend on aspects of care that might not require their special expertise. Estimates of the increased amount of care that might be provided by the appropriate utilization of well-educated PAs and NPs have ranged from 30 percent to 100 percent depending on the variables considered. Some relevant variables appear to be: (1) the type of tasks being delegated (for example, technical and repetitive versus more time-consuming comprehensive tasks); (2) the practice setting (private office, hospital, or satellite clinic, for example); (3) the number of physicians being assisted by the new professional (group versus solo practitioners); (4) the purpose for which the savings in time is utilized (for example, to increase patient load or to decrease the patient care load in order to enhance the attractiveness of a physician's practice or allow more time for continuing education for the physician); and (5) the type of patients being cared for (the well, the acutely ill, the chronically ill, the convalescent). See Judith R. Lave, Lester B. Lave, and Thomas E. Morton, "The Physician's Assistant: Exploration of the Concept," Hospitals: Journal of the American Hospital Association 45 (June 1971): pp. 46-48.

either the same fee for seeing both the physician and his assistant as would be charged for the physician's services alone[12] or a predetermined proportion of the usual fee. An instance of this latter approach was reported by Alfred Skinner who offered certain patients in his pediatric practice the opportunity to receive services from his assistant at a reduced fee; the fee charged was 0.6 units (Relative Value Study) compared with 1.5 units for a physician visit.[13]

The PA. Of the 16 respondents, 15 PA programs provided an estimate of the approximate anticipated annual salary which their graduates would earn. The salaries ranged from a low of $9000 per year to a high of $15,000 per year.* Since eight of the programs provided a range and not a specific figure, the midpoints were calculated in order to determine the median and mean expected annual salary for graduates of PA programs included in the study. On this basis, the mean and median expected salary was calculated to be $12,100 and $12,000, respectively. There was a tendency for those programs granting degrees (A.A., B.S., or M.S.) to cite a somewhat higher salary potential for their graduates than those programs awarding only a certificate.

The NP. Unfortunately, information on salary potential was not provided by a sufficient number of the NP programs to make a valid comparison between the two groups. Based on the three programs providing information, NP annual salary potential ranged from a low of less than $8000 to a high of $16,000. One program reported the results of a recent study of their graduates; two variables found to be important in affecting salary were the geographic location of the NP's employment situation and the type of agency employing her services; twenty-seven percent of their graduates earned less than $8000, 64 percent earned between $8000 and $11,000, and nine percent earned between $11,000 and $13,000.

Training Costs

Little information on a national basis is available on the cost of training either the PA or NP. Hopefully, in the near future, a cost-effectiveness analysis of national scope will be conducted to remedy the scarcity of data in this important area. Duke University's program

---

*These salary figures are comparable to those established by the Civil Service Administration in 1971. At that time, three grades were established for PAs: Grade 7 paid $8,582; Grade 9 paid $10,470; Grade 11 paid $12,615. See "Government Programs Promote Training and Use of Physicians' Assistants," American Family Physician 3, no. 5 (May 1971): 163.

reported on an in-house cost-benefit analysis; it was found that the annual training costs required to educate PAs in their program was approximately the same as that required for training medical students. Since PAs only receive two years of training, compared to the five to ten years required for medical students, the cost per PA was far below that of the physician.[14] Most cost information, to date, has consisted of "guesstimates" made by individual programs of approximate training costs per graduate. The author must also plead guilty to a similar limitation of data in this area.

The PA. Twelve of the 16 PA programs were able to provide "guesstimates" of the approximate cost of providing training on a per graduate basis. The training costs ranged from a low of $4, 500 for a two-year program (consisting of one year of didactic and one year of clinical training and awarding a master's degree upon completion) to a high of $20, 000 for a 27-month program (including two years of didactic plus a three-month preceptorship and awarding a bachelor's degree upon completion). The median figure for training costs was $11, 200. The more costly programs generally provided some stipend to their trainees, which obviously increased their estimate of average training costs.

The NP. The cost of training each NP graduate was estimated to be approximately $3, 000 for a four-month program. One of the few longer programs (18 months) reported a cost of $3, 500 per graduate. As noted in Chapter 3, the majority of early programs are only four months in length; however, they build on prior nursing education and experience which may have been acquired in a two-, three-, or four-year nursing program. Naturally, the cost of this initial investment was not included in the programs' estimates of present costs; similarly, the cost of the ex-corpsmen's prior training was not included in estimates of PA training costs.

Information on training costs per graduate PA and NP is, to date, inadequate for any valid comparison either between these two professions—or between the NP or PA and other health professionals. Estimates of costs must take into account prior investment of educational resources (cost of educational prerequisites), whether the student receives a stipend or salary while in training and from whom, and tuition costs (if any)—to name but a few of the relevant variables.

Third-Party Reimbursement

The issue of third-party reimbursement for the PAs' and NPs' services was not explicitly covered in the author's 1973 study; however, several of the programs independently noted that this issue was one of major concern for them at this time. Malcolm Todd reported in late 1972 that the AMA was involved in discussions with Medicare and other government officials to identify problems and potential solutions in this area.[15]

A major problem has arisen with regard to reimbursement of both PA and NP services under Medicare:

> The only basis in present law for coverage of the services of a physician's assistant employed by a physician is provided in section 1861 (S) (2a) and as explained in section 6103 (part B, intermediary manual), which authorizes payment for services furnished as an "incident to a physician's professional services of kinds which are commonly furnished in physicians' offices and are normally either rendered without charge or included in the physician's bill." This provision was intended to provide coverage for the traditional services of nurses, receptionists, and other assistants that are commonly furnished under the physician's personal direction in his office. The Medicare program refuses to pay for those services performed by physician's assistants (including nurse practitioners) that do not meet the definition set forth in the regulations pertaining to services incident to a physician's professional services (section 6103, part B, intermediary manual). In other words, physician-like services that are performed by nonphysician personnel outside the physician's office are not reimbursable unless the attending physician is personally present at the time these services are rendered.[16]

In an attempt to resolve this problem, Senator Gaylord Nelson (Democrat, Wisconsin) introduced an amendment to HR 1 to permit Medicare reimbursement for services rendered by assistants to physicians both in and outside physician's offices whether or not the supervising physician is personally present at the time the services are given. The amendment would also have required that assistants be licensed or certified in their respective states and that the supervising physician would assume full liability for the actions of his employee. However, the Senate Finance Committee modified Senator Nelson's amendment to allow Medicare reimbursement for PA and NP services only in experimental projects. HEW was to conduct demonstration projects to determine "equitable" levels of payment for such services. A broader interpretation of section 6103 is not expected until ". . . there are greater numbers of physician's assistants and nurse practitioners in actual practice and sufficient data concerning cost benefit and patient acceptance has been collected to warrant a policy change."[17]

The issue of third-party reimbursement for PA and NP services is not limited to the governmental arena. Private non-profit health insurance plans (for example, Blue Shield and Blue Cross) have shown an equal unwillingness to pioneer in this area. As of 1971, Judith Lave et al. reported that Blue Shield would not pay for obstetrical care provided by a qualified nurse-midwife.[18] In order to maximize efficiency in the actual use of the NP and the PA as an added incentive to widely employ these new professionals, problems of reimbursement must be resolved as soon as possible. If PA and NP services are not eligible for third-party reimbursement, the entire costs of their employment would be necessarily assumed by their employers; this would result in higher costs to the consumer as well as possibly encouraging the maldistribution of these new professionals. For example, PAs and NPs may find employment opportunities primarily in large urban financially lucrative practices; such a distribution would do little to correct the specialty and geographic maldistribution problems previously noted.*

STRUCTURAL DEVELOPMENT OF THE EARLY PROGRAMS

The PA. As an educational program matures, goals, objectives, curricula, and the like are constantly subjected to evaluation and reformulation. The early PA programs had undergone a number of changes in both philosophy and content in the period between 1970 and 1973. These changes were reflected most often in curriculum revisions. In addition, some programs reported basic changes in their perceptions of the type of PA they were attempting to educate—in terms of both function and ideological orientation of the new professional.

Some curriculum changes were very specific; that is, they dealt with particular course additions and deletions to program content. For example, one program had added courses in general medicine, pathology, applied physiology, obstetrics, and psychiatry and had omitted courses in biomedical physics. Most saw curriculum revision in more abstract terms; the desire was to develop broad-based core curricula—generally increasing the clinical component while

---

*That the employment of a PA or a NP is economically feasible even in a rural group practice setting was skillfully illustrated recently by Regina McCormack and Charles Miller. A computer simulation model of a hypothetical rural group practice was constructed; utilizing data from a rural community in central Virginia and a local fee schedule, the simulation demonstrated the economic viability of rural group practice and indicated that the use of an assistant (in this case, a primary care nurse) to provide care to a certain proportion of the patients enhanced both the economic efficiency and financial attractiveness of the practice. See Regina C. McCormack and Charles W. Miller, "The Economic Feasibility of Rural Group Practice: Influence of Non-Physician Practitioners in Primary Care," Medical Care 10, no. 1 (January-February 1972): 73-80.

simultaneously adopting more of a liberal arts orientation. As noted previously, 14 of the 16 early PA programs now educate primary care PAs; three of these 14 programs had originally educated specialists; since 1970, they had revised their curricula in order to emphasize the education of generalists while retaining specialty options to be pursued after completion of the core courses. Two programs, originally stressing the institution as a work setting for their specialist PAs, now educate only primary care PAs to work in the community.

Several programs had interesting developmental patterns that are worthy of special comment. One program had begun as a tuition-free demonstration project, with private foundation funding, recruiting indigenous low-status health workers. The program had been based in a medical center and had awarded a certificate upon completion of the course of study. By 1973, it had become an official tuition program (tuition waivers were still available) sponsored by both an academic institution and a medical center. It now offered two alternative routes to a PA certificate, one awarding an A. A. degree and the other granting a B. S. degree. The former was designed as a route encouraging the recruitment of lower level health workers (for example, corpsmen and licensed practical nurses); credit from one program could be easily applied toward advanced entry into the higher degree program. The clinical portion of both programs was similar; however, those who chose the B. S. program received more academic work in the biological and medical sciences; credit from this program could be applied toward a higher degree (for example, an M. D.).

A second PA program, placing substantial importance on career mobility for the PA, had been one of the early advocates of a liberal education for this emerging health professional. The program had clearly defined its goals and objectives long before the first class had been admitted in 1968. Flexibility was built into the original program so that changes in curriculum could be easily effected. In 1973, they reported that the curriculum had been revised in numerous ways (for example, addition of psychiatry and omission of physics) in order to reflect the changing needs of the PA role as they and their graduates perceived it. The curriculum had three distinct facets: (1) selected medical courses; (2) selected non-medical courses in the natural and social sciences; and (3) selected full time clinical experiences with different preceptorships in a variety of settings (for example, hospital, clinic, school of medicine, and private office). The successful candidate was granted a B. S. in Medical Sciences; with this degree, one could pursue further graduate studies in the sciences or enter medical school.

Two of the programs, having initially invested substantial money and time in intensive task analyses of their respective types of PAs, had had to make few changes in their programs. As planned, one had introduced an audio-tutorial self-study approach for the first phase of its basic curriculum. The other program had increased the length of the training period by several months and now spent more time in clinical practice than had been originally anticipated. Still a third program's initial intensive efforts to plan thoroughly had been rewarded by sustained active support for its program, particularly in its immediate service area. They had used a collaborative planning model—actively involving groups with vested interests in the program from the very beginning; meetings were held with practicing physicians, organized medicine, medical school faculty, the state nursing association, state hospitals, and drug associations. The program's staff and physician-preceptors met with local leaders in preceptor communities before the PA's arrival. The program had used an involvement planning approach to develop the actual curriculum; they confronted and solved problems as they arose with all interested parties—students, faculty, preceptors—taking part in the ultimate solution.

In sum, between 1970 and 1973, there were some definite changes in the PA programs' perception of the PA role. This was reflected in large measure in curriculum changes. The PA was no longer seen as a technician, an office assistant, or a narrow specialist. An emphasis was placed on his role as a primary health care provider. Although the dependence of the role was still stressed, professional qualities of intelligence, code of ethics, ability to relate to people, capacity for reasoned judgments both in emergencies and in routine care situations, and a service orientation were of the utmost importance. Attention had been given to providing the PA with a broader, more liberal education, and thus hopefully providing him with greater opportunities for career mobility. As one program aptly stated, the PA of 1973 should no longer be considered a technician—he is a new health professional.

The NP. The early NP programs had also undergone changes as their programs matured. Curriculum revisions were noted by most of the programs. As well as specific course additions, more emphasis was placed on techniques of physical assessment, on counseling and interviewing skills, on approaches to meeting the psychosocial needs of patients and their families in the community setting, and on providing students with more relevant comprehensive clinical experiences. One program was in the process of integrating the NP role into the basic nursing curriculum on the baccalaureate level. Another had integrated some of their NP training with that of the medical students and residents within the medical center; in this manner, new life had been given to the concept of a team approach to health care and mutual respect for each member's unique competencies was promoted.

Role definition had been a problem experienced by many of the NP students. Attempts were made to provide students with NP role-models in institutions, offices, and outpatient settings. Opportunities were found to allow the NP student to assume considerable independent responsibility for comprehensive care regardless of her student status.

Most programs had not changed their basic philosophy. They were educating professional nurses to assume expanded roles as primary health care providers. The team approach to health care was still actively promoted. The NP was to be considered an essential part of that team—a coequal with any of the other participants. She was a health professional in her own right who collaborated with others on the health team in order to provide the best care possible to her patients. Above all, she was to be the patient's advocate—both providing care herself and making the system manageable to the patient.

CONCLUDING REMARKS

The focus of this chapter has been on the evolutionary development of the PA concept between 1970 and late 1973. Much progress had been made in that period toward resolving some of the basic issues confronting this new health provider. The PA was to be considered a new health professional—not merely a dependent appendage of the physician. Although not licensed, national certification examinations have given an aura of legitimacy to the PA and promoted his geographic mobility. As noted in Chapter 4, steps have been taken to encourage the PA's legal use in all types of health care settings—including the hospital.

Two major issues still remain the source of considerable debate: (1) the role of the PA vis-a-vis other nonphysician health professionals (with particular reference to the registered nurse and the NP); and (2) the effect of third-party reimbursement on utilization potential. The educators of the PA and the NP appear cognizant of the unique qualities of each of their respective professionals. However, at this point, it appears that the NP programs perceive greater differences between NPs and PAs than do the PA programs! An attempt was made in this chapter to reflect the distinct attributes of each of these health professionals and the unique problems each must face.

One would hope that the wasteful paradox now existing in the reimbursement area would be resolved quickly. At a time when many governmental and private agencies are actively supporting both the PA and the NP, positive governmental and private third-party reimbursement policies for these new providers are lacking. The policies are actually inhibiting the innovative use of these providers in new service areas. Ever greater financial support must be given both the programs and the practitioners in these new fields.

The following chapter presents the results of a local case study conducted by the author. Specifically, the receptivity of one community of health professionals and patients to the anticipated introduction of the PA is examined.

NOTES

1. American Nurses' Association and American Academy of Pediatrics, "Guidelines on Short-Term Continuing Education Programs for Pediatric Nurse Associates," mimeographed (New York: Division on Maternal and Child Health Nursing, American Nurses' Association, January 29, 1971), pp. 1-7.

2. Ibid., p. 3.

3. Irene Turner et al., "Evaluation of the Nurse Associate in a Variety of Health Care Settings," mimeographed (Chicago: Rush Presbyterian-St. Luke's Medical Center, September 1973), p. 8.

4. "Evaluation Report: Pediatric Nurse Associate Project," mimeographed (Augusta, Maine: Regional Medical Program, January 1972), pp. 1-11.

5. Turner, op. cit., pp. 1-8.

6. National Academy of Sciences, *New Members of the Physician's Health Team: Physician's Assistants* (Washington, D.C.: The Academy, 1970), p. 3.

7. "Model Legislation Project for Physician's Assistants," mimeographed (Durham, North Carolina: Department of Community Health Sciences, Duke University, August 1972), pp. 1-60.

8. Ibid., pp. 31-43.

9. Ibid., pp. 31-38.

10. Ibid., pp. 41-43.

11. Ibid., pp. 38-40.

12. Donald W. Schiff, Charles H. Fraser, and Heather L. Walters, "The Pediatric Nurse Practitioner in the Office of Pediatricians in Private Practice," *Pediatrics* 44, no. 1 (July 1969): 66.

13. Alfred L. Skinner, "Parental Acceptance of Delegated Pediatric Services," *Pediatrics* 41, no. 5 (May 1968): 1003-1004.

14. D. Robert Howard and Emil Fasser, "Duke University's Physician's Assistant Program," *Hospital Progress*, February 1970, p. 51.

15. Malcolm C. Todd, "Medical Manpower and the Emergence of New Professions," *Texas Medicine* 68, no. 10 (October 1972): 60-64.

16. Ibid., p. 64.

17. Ibid.

18. Judith R. Lave, Lester B. Lave, and Thomas E. Morton, "The Physician's Assistant: Exploration of a Concept," *Hospitals: Journal of the American Hospital Association* 45 (June 1971): 48.

CHAPTER

6

THE OBSTETRICAL PHYSICIAN'S ASSISTANT: A LOCAL CASE STUDY

INTRODUCTION

In this chapter the results of the 1970 local case study are presented. The data are analyzed and the findings presented herein in a straightforward format without extensive discussion or speculation. Concluding remarks and broader implications of the local study as well as the two national surveys are reserved for Chapter 7. At the end of this chapter, a series of working hypotheses derived from the local study are given. The analysis is otherwise centered around the responses of the three groups surveyed: patients, physicians, and nurses; as previously cited (Chapter 2), a particularly high response rate was obtained for each of the respondent groups. A fourth section is devoted to an obstetrical task analysis.

THE PATIENTS

The patient group in the study community—a medium-sized Southern city—comprised 45 expectant mothers. Approximately one-third were patients at a local hospital outpatient clinic, while two-thirds received obstetrical services from private physicians. Fifty-eight percent were white and 42 percent were blacks. The majority were between the ages of 18 and 25 (64 percent); 9 percent were under 18, and 27 percent were over 25 years of age. With respect to education, the largest number of women had either less than a high school education (27 percent) or had at least some college (42 percent); 18 percent completed high school and nine percent had had more than four years of college. Twenty-seven percent (12) of the expectant mothers were college students at the time of the study. Of the 31 women who gave their husband's occupation, 51 percent (16) of the husbands were college students; 15 of the remaining 16 husbands were employed in professional or managerial type jobs. Only 13 percent were originally from a home town not in the South. Excluding eight nonrespondents, 84 percent were experiencing their first pregnancy. Approximately 14 percent of the women were in the first trimester, 43 percent in the second trimester, and another 43 percent were in their third trimester of pregnancy. In a demographic sense, then, the expectant mothers studied appeared to possess substantial heterogeneity; such heterogeneity suggests that it is more likely than not that the patient group was fairly representative of the patients in the wider community.

Of the women reporting, 84 percent (38) stated that they would be willing to use the services of an obstetrical PA while only 7 percent (3) stated they would not; 9 percent (4) were undecided. Acknowledging the difficulty of evaluating affirmative responses to the use of a new (and for this group, unfamiliar) type of health worker, a number of follow-up questions attempted to elicit how acceptable this new type of worker would be. Identifying the tasks women were willing to have the PA perform should more accurately reflect the degree of acceptance which the PA might anticipate; that is, if they would use him for tasks ordinarily deemed to belong exclusively to the physician, this would indicate considerable acceptability; however, if they would use him only for tasks presently delegated to allied health workers (for example, laboratory technicians) their acceptance of this new health provider role should probably be considered minimal. Table 6.1 indicates what tasks women would, or would not, be willing to have the obstetrical PA provide for them in the physician's office.

The tasks which the patients were most readily willing to delegate to the obstetrical PA (recording blood pressure and conducting urine tests and blood tests) are already delegated by the physicians to other health workers. Although only nine (20 percent) were wiling to have the PA do a physical examination that includes a pelvic examination, 26 (58 percent) were willing to have the PA do an initial physical without a pelvic examination. Evaluating the fetal heartbeat and assessing position of the fetus as well as answering general questions about their pregnancy were tasks a substantial percentage of the women felt comfortable about being delegated to an obstetrical PA. Although only a small percentage were willing to have an initial pelvic examination done by the PA, a sizeable percentage of the expectant mothers would allow him to do the tasks that comprise the majority of visits a woman makes to an obstetrician during her pregnancy.

The ultimate degree of acceptance of an obstetrical PA should be allowing him to deliver a woman's baby. One of the questions addressed itself to this issue. See Table 6.2. Given the untested nature of the obstetrical PA role, it is surprising that only 44 percent would not allow a PA to deliver their babies. One may question whether the 38 percent who said they would allow the PA to deliver

TABLE 6.1

Tasks Patients Would Permit the Obstetrical PA to Perform

Tasks	Yes %	Yes (f)	No %	No (f)	No Response %	No Response (f)
Initial physical exam. including pelvic exam.	20	(9)	76	(34)	4	(2)
Initial physical exam. excluding pelvic exam.	58	(26)	38	(17)	4	(2)
Blood pressure	94	(42)	2	(1)	4	(2)
Urine test	85	(38)	11	(5)	4	(2)
Check fetal heartbeat	67	(30)	29	(13)	4	(2)
Check position and size of fetus (by feeling abdomen)	47	(21)	49	(22)	4	(2)
Blood test	89	(40)	7	(3)	4	(2)
Answer questions about problems in pregnancy	42	(19)	54	(24)	4	(2)

Source: Compiled by the author.

TABLE 6.2

Opinions Regarding Delivery by the PA

Q. Would you be willing to have a trained PA deliver your baby? (Assume that your doctor has previously examined you and assured you that your delivery would be a normal one.)

Yes, but only if my doctor is present		Yes. Doctor need not be present		No		No Response	
%	(f)	%	(f)	%	(f)	%	(f)
38	(17)	16	(7)	44	(20)	2	(1)

Source: Compiled by the author.

their babies only if the physician were also present, were really exhibiting confidence in the new health professional. It is certainly questionable whether allowing delivery only with this limitation would result in a more efficient use of the physicians' time. However, viewing this finding in a positive fashion, at least 38 percent were willing to allow the PA to perform a task that has been in recent times, at least in most parts of this country, an almost sacrosanct function of the physician. Perhaps, with exposure to the new professional, some of this group would be willing to allow the PA to deliver their babies without the physician being present.

When level of education was introduced as a control, there appeared few, if any, strong relationships between levels of formal education and degree of acceptance. All women, regardless of years of schooling, were favorable toward the concept and general use of the PA, although there was a very slight tendency for this receptivity to be positively related to education. Upon examining crucial obstetrical tasks which the PA might perform, there appeared to be somewhat of a difference between groups; while 35 percent (17) of those with a high school education or less said they would allow a PA to do the initial physical examination, including the pelvic, none of those with more than a college education agreed to this task delegation. In this instance, tolerance seems to drop off as the education of the respondent increases. Perhaps the most crucial task for the obstetrician, or his PA, is that of the delivery. Here the data show little convincing evidence of a definite relationship between willingness to have the PA deliver the baby and the level of education of the respondent. However, the data were slightly suggestive of the possible existence of a curvilinear relationship between education and the acceptance of the PA delivering the baby (with or without the obstetrician present). Acceptance seemed to be greatest in the group with the least education (12 years or less) and for those with the most education (more than four years of college). Least acceptance was evidenced in the middle-range group: women with some college or those who had completed college.

When term of pregnancy was examined as a control, it was found that the farther a woman was into her pregnancy, the less receptive she was to the PA. Women in their third trimester were less receptive to the use of the PA in principle and in terms of specific task delegation. For example, 58 percent (11) of those in their third trimester would oppose the use of the obstetrical PA to deliver their babies regardless if the physician were present or not; only 37 percent (7) of those in the second trimester would oppose such delegation.

One of the advantages often cited for the introduction of a PA is that it may help curb the rising cost of health care. The patients were asked what effect (if any) a possible cost reduction would have on their willingness to use the PA's services. Table 6.3 presents the results. A review of Table 6.3 confirms the belief that a reduction in

TABLE 6.3

Effect of Cost on Potential Patient Usage of the PA

Q. If, by using the services of a PA the total cost of your care during pregnancy, labor, and delivery were reduced, would you be more willing to use the services of the PA?

Yes		Yes, but it depends on the amount of reduction.		No, cost not important. Would use PA.		No, cost not important. Would not use PA.		No Response	
%	(f)	%	(f)	%	(f)	%	(f)	%	(f)
53	(24)	18	(8)	20	(9)	7	(3)	2	(1)

Source: Compiled by the author.

cost of obstetrical care would promote the utilization of the obstetrical PA. As noted, only 3 women (7 percent) stated they would not use the PA under any circumstances while 9 (20 percent) would use the PA even if there were no reduction in cost. The relationship between cost and usage held when education and when term of pregnancy were introduced: (1) reduction in cost was the most important for the least educated group and least important as a consideration by the middle-range educated group; (2) regardless of the term of pregnancy, a reduction in cost would make the use of a PA more acceptable to women.

The registered nurse was most often selected as the preferred recruitment source for the obstetrical PA. Forty-nine percent (22) of the respondents preferred this source. The reasons most frequently cited for this preference were that the RN was already an accepted health provider and she had more relevant educational preparation and practical experience than the others listed as potential recruitment sources. (The list included the ex-military medical corpsman as a possible choice.) The second recruitment source most often selected was the college graduate with a health-related major such as biology. It is interesting to note that neither sex was favored over the other for use as an obstetrical PA. Sixty-four percent of the respondents (29) did not have a preference for sex for the role of PA. Only 13 percent (6) preferred a female, while 20 percent (9) preferred a male.

While 53 percent (24) felt that there was a job for both the PA and the nurse in the obstetrician's office, few were able to differentiate their respective potential roles. Sixteen percent (7) felt that the PA, with his special training, should directly assist the doctor with his tasks and utilize the nurse to help him; they suggested the assistant could do counseling while the nurse could perform routine tasks such as checking blood pressure, making urine tests, and so on. Only two expectant mothers suggested that the nurse could work more closely with the doctor and the patient and the PA could deal with the more technical office patient care tasks. Another three women (seven percent) felt that the assistant would "replace" the physician, not the nurse; as such, the nurse could "continue with her regular duties"; however, no patient was able to adequately define what the nurse's duties were, or should be, in the obstetrician's office. An additional nine percent (4) felt that, providing the PA was a male, a female nurse should be present to help her prepare for examinations.

What was the most important advantage patients saw in the use of an obstetrical PA? Forty-two percent of the respondents said that, because the doctor would be less burdened with routine care, he would have more time to spend caring for particular problems patients might have during their pregnancies. An additional 22 percent (10) felt that the PA could fill a need they experienced for someone to talk with them about minor problems and general questions they had about their pregnancies.

The most important disadvantage which the women felt might occur if PAs were employed by their physician was the fear that, because the doctor would be able to increase the total number of patients he sees, they would never have an opportunity to see the physician unless they had a serious problem; 38 percent (17) cited this as a potential disadvantage. Other disadvantages mentioned were: (1) a fear of receiving inferior care (20 percent); (2) a fear the PA would miss certain medical problems until they had become very serious (16 percent); and (3) a feeling that they would not be able to discuss very personal problems with someone other than their own physician (9 percent). A fear of receiving inferior care was most often cited by the least educated women. None of the women with the most education cited this possible disadvantage.

Ninety-one percent (41) of the expectant mothers felt that there was definitely a shortage of obstetricians in the community. The vast majority complained of having to wait a long time for an initial appointment and of feeling that the doctor was terribly rushed when they did see him. One mother commented, "My doctor never really takes the time to answer my questions. If you don't know what questions to ask, you would never find out anything about your pregnancy." Despite the fact that women complained about the shortage of obstetricians, 37 percent (17) said that they were basically satisfied with the care they received. Fifteen percent (7) were disturbed about the doctor being too rushed and another 15 percent felt that they saw too many doctors, which made care too impersonal.

Although the traditional view of the doctor as a "miracle worker" appears to be dying out, still 15 women emphasized their personal need to view the physician as a friend or father-image. Sixty-eight percent (37) of the respondents viewed the doctor as a highly educated professional who is able to help them with their health needs. When asked to further typify their feeling toward what a physician should be, 40 percent (18) emphasized competency and 31 percent (14) emphasized the need to show personal concern for them as individuals.

THE PHYSICIANS

The physician group consisted of seven specialists in obstetrics and gynecology, five of whom predominately practice obstetrics and two of whom have recently limited their practices to gynecology; the eighth member of this group was a general practitioner who maintains a substantial obstetrical practice. Seventy-five percent (6) of the physicians obtained their medical training in a southern state. Five cited a southern town as their home town while two originally came from the North or North Central portion of the United States. Four had practiced in the community for less than ten years while the other four had practiced there from 14 to 23 years. Three were between 30 and 40 years of age while the eldest was in his mid-fifties.

As practicing obstetricians, all but one saw a local need for at least one of the three types of PAs (as defined by the 1970 National Academy of Sciences' report). Six stated they would use a PA in their practices if one were available for employment in the area. Of the two who would not use a PA, one felt no need for a PA in his personal practice, and the second felt that the use of PAs was not yet justified—his value in medicine had not yet been proven. Excluding the two physicians who would not use a PA, 84 percent (5) would be willing to be the first obstetrician in the community to employ such an assistant. Although the vast majority saw a need for and would use a PA in the community, only one felt the shortage of obstetricians in the area sufficiently acute to be considered of crisis proportions. The one physician who perceived an acute shortage of obstetricians had already limited his practice to gynecology!

One-half of the physicians ranked the physician's associate (Type A) as being potentially the most useful type of PA for their needs and 38 percent (3) ranked the specialist assistant (Type B) most useful. The rationale most often cited for their choice was that this type of assistant would prove most effective and be more content in a dependent "assistant-type" position. The second reason most often mentioned was that their choice had "sufficient relevant education."

The development of a new type of health worker, particularly one who would exercise some independent medical judgment, is always surrounded by questions regarding potential legal difficulties. Seventy-five percent (6) of the physicians favored licensure for the PA. Essentially, the reason given for favoring licensure was that the license would provide a "policing" function over the PA; licensure would provide minimum standards and these, in turn, would control the education and practice of the PA. One physician, who did not favor licensure, felt that the licensed PA might become too independent; an organization of licensed PAs might become "like a union."

Although licensure was favored by three out of four physicians, only half felt that any professional liability problems resulting from the use of the PA would be resolved by the PA being completely responsible for his own actions. Three felt that the physician would remain responsible for the PA's actions under the doctrine of respondeat superior. Even if PAs were to become licensed, only 25 percent (2) felt that a licensed PA would be able to be hired by hospitals, such as nurses are today, under the auspices of the hospital's medical board.

It is interesting to note the type of individual the obstetricians felt should be recruited for the obstetrical PA in 1970. Eighty-eight percent (7) favored the recruitment of registered nurses while only 13 percent (1) favored ex-military corpsmen. The rationale most often given (50 percent of the respondents) for choosing the RN was that she was already a health worker who is accepted by both the public and by the physician. Twenty-five percent (2) felt the RN would be the best recruitment source because she was the most likely to train for and be content in an "assistant" type of occupation. When informed of a recent ANA-NLN joint statement (October 1970) disapproving of the use of the RN as a PA, five out of eight obstetricians disagreed with the ANA-NLN. Several reasons were given for their disagreement: the nurse was the only "logical" choice, she was already being used in many medical assistant-type roles (for example, nurse anesthetist), and since she does so little actual nursing now, being an obstetrical assistant would not take her away from actual nursing! They suggested training more nurses and in particular increasing the nurse's salary in order to entice more people into nursing; therefore, if some nurses took "a modest amount of additional training" to become PAs, the total nursing complement would not be reduced.

None of the physicians were aware of the recent AMA position on medicine and nursing which had been published in the Journal of the American Medical Association in September, 1970.[1] The only professional organization that they felt would be of particular relevance to them in helping them clarify their opinions concerning the practice of medicine in general, and toward the obstetrical PA in particular, was the American College of Obstetricians and Gynecologists.* This

---

*Interestingly, shortly after the local study was completed, the American College of Obstetricians and Gynecologists, the Nurses' Association of the American College of Obstetricians and Gynecologists, and the American College of Nurse-Midwives issued a joint statement on methods of improving the availability and quality of maternity care. The statement, issued on January 14, 1971, called

organization was named by 75 percent (6) of the physicians while the American Medical Association was only named by one physician as personally influencing him in medical matters. Membership in non-medical community organizations was minimal; no physician presently held a leadership role outside of the study community. The faction that they felt would be most influential in promoting the acceptability of the PA concept was neither the AMA nor the public. It was the individual physicians by their expressed demand.

Most of the physicians favored the RN for the new position of obstetrical PA. However, whether or not the nurse is in fact recruited for the PA role, what effect did they feel the PA would have upon the position of the nurse who currently works with the obstetrician? Eighty-eight percent agreed that their present nurse assistants were "indispensable and adequately trained." However, 50 percent (4) added that they would be even more helpful if they had more specialized training before employment. Fifty percent felt that the new job of PA could provide a career ladder for the nurse in obstetrics by providing her with just a little more training; 50 percent also felt that the new job could possibly interfere with the present physician-nurse relationship in that the obstetrical PA may, in effect, be an additional boss for whom the obstetrical nurse would have to work. Twenty-five percent (2) felt that the new job might prove to be competitive with the nurse's present role in obstetrics; 38 percent felt that the tasks that may be lost to the obstetrical nurse are tasks which never should have been delegated to her; that is, they are medical tasks that have fallen by default to the nurse because obstetricians have become too busy to handle them themselves. However, if the tasks delegated to the PA would take away all or most of the functions now given the nurse, 63 percent (5) would not favor it. Only 25 percent (2) felt that such an occurrence would be desirable in order to free the obstetrical nurse to work in other areas of nursing where she may be needed more than in obstetrics.

All medical costs are rising rapidly—obstetrical costs are no exception. The introduction of new types of health professionals into the provision of health care has been suggested as one way to curb these rising costs. Accordingly, the obstetricians were asked what effect they felt the use of obstetrical PAs would have upon the cost of obstetrical care. The physicians studied were clearly divided in their opinions concerning the effect of employing obstetrical PAs on the cost of care; 38 percent (3) felt it would reduce the cost of obstetrical care to the patient, another 38 percent (3) felt it would have no effect upon cost, and 25 percent (2) felt it would increase costs.

---

for the formation of teams of physicians, nurse-midwives, obstetrical nurses, and other health personnel. See Eleanor C. Lambertsen, "Not Quite MD, More Than PA," Hospitals: Journal of the American Hospital Association 45 (December 1971): 72-73.

The rationale given for reduction in cost was essentially that the PA would be able to supply a substantial portion of the obstetrical care given to patients with few if any complications; these patients would receive care at a lower total cost than presently possible. Those who felt it would have no effect upon the cost of obstetrical care to the patient argued that although more patients would be served and thus more income would be realized, the salary of the PA would offset the greater income so that obstetrical costs would remain essentially the same. Those who felt that the cost of obstetrical care would increase felt that: (1) their individual patients would be getting more care and therefore would be willing to pay more for it; and (2) the added cost of the PA's salary would necessitate the physician charging more for care.

The physicians saw two major advantages for the use of obstetrical PAs. His use would enable the physician to provide more care to greater numbers of patients and would free the physician of much routine care in order that he might spend more time on those patients who most need his care (that is, the obstetrical patient with complications). Approximately 50 percent (4) of the physicians stressed these two advantages. Only two physicians felt that the use of an obstetrical PA was potentially disadvantageous; they felt it might become a "back door" into the practice of medicine and could, if improperly used, reduce the closeness of the physician-patient relationship.

Because there was some concern for the effect of the PA upon the delivery of obstetrical care, it was interesting to note the characteristics which the physicians felt should be ideally possessed by "the good doctor," "the good nurse," and "the good patient." Fifty percent (4) stressed the need for intellectual competence as being the physician's most important attribute; the remaining 50 percent stressed the need for honesty by the physician in his dealings with his patients and an ability to empathize with them. Efficiency and competency were rated as the most important attributes of a good nurse by 50 percent; the remaining 50 percent stressed the need to be genuinely concerned with the patients' welfare. The characteristics that 75 percent (6) of the physicians felt "the good patient" should possess emphasized efficiency of health care; that is, three felt that "carrying out the doctor's orders faithfully" was most important and three felt that asking relevant questions and answering questions with relevant answers was most important in the ideal patient. Only one physician stressed the need for patients to report health problems promptly as being characteristic of "the good patient."

As previously noted, 88 percent of the obstetricians saw a need for an obstetrical PA and 75 percent stated that they would employ one (if available) in their practice; such a positive response could be interpreted as a mandate for the introduction of an obstetrical PA. However, before drawing this conclusion, it is important to know what potential role the PA would fulfill—what specific tasks are the obstetricians willing to delegate to such a health worker? It is perhaps equally important to first note what tasks are now being delegated and to be aware of the opinions of those who presently perform many of these tasks: the obstetrical nurses. After summarizing the results of the nurse respondents, a tabular analysis of present and potential delegation of obstetrical patient care tasks is presented.

THE NURSES

There were 40 nurses included in the study: 23 registered nurses (RNs) and 17 practical nurses (LPNs).* Of the RNs, 14 (61 percent) received their basic nursing education in a diploma program, eight (35 percent) received their bachelor's degree in nursing and one received an associate of arts degree in nursing. Only two (9 percent) had received some formal postgraduate education in obstetrics. Eight (20 percent) were employed by the obstetricians in their office practice while the remaining 32 (80 percent) worked in the obstetrical services (labor, delivery, and postpartum) of the two local general hospitals. Only one LPN was employed as an office nurse; the rest of the LPNs worked in the two general hospitals. Of the total nurse group 30 percent were black and 70 percent were white; all were female. Twenty-eight percent (11) were under the age of 26, 60 percent (24) were between 26 and 50 years of age, and 10 percent (4) over 50. Sixty-five percent (26) had worked in obstetrics between six and ten years while the remaining 17.5 percent (7) had worked in obstetrics for 11 to 25 years. Approximately 88 percent of the LPNs and 60 percent of the RNs originally came from a southern state. All of the LPNs received their nursing education in the study community or elsewhere in the state; only 43 percent of the RNs had done so.

As practicing obstetrical nurses, 88 percent (35) saw a need for at least one of the types of PAs (as defined by the Board on Medicine of the National Academy of Sciences) to work in the obstetrical field. Sixty-three percent (25) felt that the physician's associate (Type A)

---

*The local study attempted to survey opinions among all obstetrical nurses in the community. The practical nurses provide a substantial portion of that care; therefore, it was felt that in order to obtain an accurate reflection of the receptivity of the obstetrical nurse to the possible introduction of an obstetrical PA, the nursing group should include both LPNs and RNs. Most of the discussion will focus on the attitudes of the total nursing group; only where LPNs and RNs displayed substantially different attitudes will the two groups be differentiated.

would be most useful, whereas the nonspecialized assistant (Type C) was rated the least useful. Self-reliance was rated (by 50 percent) as one of the most important characteristics for the obstetrical PA to possess; also important were the PA's ability to complement and not compete with the nurse's role in obstetrics, as well as his willingness to be content to function in an assistant capacity. Thirty-five percent (4) felt that the latter two characteristics were particularly relevant. Although 84 percent (5) of the physicians had stated they would be willing to be the first obstetrician in the community to employ an obstetrical PA, only 33 percent of the nurses felt they would be willing to train for, and then function as, one of the first obstetrical PAs in the community. The remainder were equally divided being being undecided about pursuing such a role and definitely being opposed to assuming such a role. Approximately one-third of both the RNs and LPNs would consult a physician in helping them to form their opinion toward an obstetrical PA; 53 percent (12) of the RNs would consult fellow staff nurses while 53 percent (9) of the LPNs would consult a nurse in a supervisory position. Relevant practical experience, not friendship or advanced education, was given as the reason for selecting a fellow nurse, supervisor, or doctor with respect to this issue.

With regard to resolution of potential legal difficulties often encountered in the development of a new type of health professional, the nurses were essentially in agreement with the physicians. As the physicians had strongly endorsed licensure for the PA, so did the nurses; 85 percent (34) favored licensure for the PA in order to maintain minimum standards of education and practice. Six (15 percent) did not favor licensure at the moment; however, they felt it would be useful in the future. Two of the six were fearful that the PA might become "too independent" if he obtained his own license. Ninety-eight percent (39) felt that PAs would inevitably become licensed.

Although licensure was favored by 85 percent of the nurses, only 35 percent (14) felt that any professional liability problems would be resolved by the PA becoming completely responsible for his own actions. Another 35 percent felt that the physician would retain considerable professional liability for the action of a PA even if the latter had his own license. (In this assumption of physician liability, the nurses apparently envisioned the PA's legal status to be equivalent to their own.) Whereas only 25 percent (2) of the obstetricians felt that professional organizations (such as the AMA), with their political influence, would be most influential in resolving the legal difficulties concerning the use of the PA, 50 percent of the nurses felt this would be the case. (It is interesting to note that in this regard the nurses viewed the AMA as having more influence than the physicians apparently felt the AMA possessed.)

There were only slight differences of opinion among the RNs and LPNs with regard to what type of individual should be recruited for the position of PA. Seventy percent (28) of the total number of nurses preferred the RN as the first recruitment source: this represented 65 percent (11) of the LPNs and 74 percent (17) of the RNs. More than one-half of the RNs felt that college graduates with a health-related major or ex-military corpsmen were also good choices to become PAs. More than one-half of the LPNs selected the college graduate with a health-related major, but only 30 percent (5) selected the corpsman. Thirty-one percent (7) of the RNs felt LPNs could take additional training to become PAs while 47 percent (8) of the LPNs mentioned this choice. The rationale most often mentioned by both RNs and LPNs for their preferred recruitment choice (the RN) was that this individual was already a health professional accepted by both the public and by other health professionals. This opinion was in accord with that given by the physicians for their recruitment choice. The RNs most often stressed the need for sufficient health-related educational background as an additional rationale for their selection (35 percent) while the LPNs stressed the likelihood of their preferred recruitment source to be willing to train for an "assistant" type of occupation (24 percent). Although there was a slight tendency for the RNs to favor females for the role of obstetrical PA and for the LPNs to favor males for the role, overwhelmingly (73 percent) both RNs and LPNs felt that either sex should be equally acceptable in the job of PA. This contrasted sharply with the physicians, 75 percent of whom definitely favored the female to act in the role of the PA. The nurses' opinion, in this regard, was more akin to the patient group.

The nurses were informed of the AMA's recent (September 1970) official position on "Nursing and Medicine in the 70's" which, in essence, supported the role of the nurse as the PA.[2] Eighty percent (32) agreed with the position; 65 percent (26) agreed completely while 5 percent felt only on-the-job training was needed as opposed to the AMA's suggested "modest amount of additional formal training." Of the eight nurses (20 percent) who disagreed, only one did so because she felt that there were too few nurses now and therefore, the PA should be taken from nonnursing areas. The remaining seven (five of whom were RNs) disagreed because they felt that a "modest amount of additional formal training" would not be sufficient for the nurse to assume this new role; in essence, they felt that the nurse's role has been too dependent a role, and, thus, to become a PA, the nurse would have to go through extensive role reorientation.

The ANA and NLN had recently (late 1970) issued statements regarding their official position on the proper role of the nurse in relation to the PA.[3] In essence, these positions stated that nurses are needed for nursing; nursing schools are not for the training of the PA. The response of the nurses to this position was very interesting. Only 24 percent (4) of the LPNs and 9 percent (2) of the RNs agreed completely with the ANA-NLN positions. However, an additional 53 percent (9) of the LPNs and 43 percent (10) of the RNs agreed with the ANA-NLN with the exception that agreeing with the position did not negate the use of the RN as a PA; that is, they did not feel nursing schools should train PAs and yet saw nothing incongruous in suggesting a special program (outside the nursing school) that a nurse could enroll in to become a PA once she had completed her basic nursing studies. The remaining RNs (43 percent) disagreed with the ANA-NLN position. Two reasons were frequently given: (1) it is up to the individual nurse to decide if she wants further education; and (2) nurses are trained for many areas of health care, not only bedside nursing; they are being used in many areas other than nursing care per se (for example, nurse anesthetist) and so should be able to become PAs if they choose.

When nurses who chose the nurse as the preferred recruitment source were asked how they would resolve any conflict which might arise from their choice and the official position of the ANA and NLN, 50 percent (20) did not feel there was any real conflict to be resolved. Although nursing schools should not train PAs, the individual nurse has the right (after completion of a nursing program) to continue her education "in any way she sees fit." Thirteen percent (5) agreed that the nurse with PA training should probably no longer be considered a nurse; however, in her new role, she would be contributing to good patient care which is the "only important issue at stake."

The only professional organizations mentioned as being considered relevant to the individual nurses in helping them clarify their general opinions regarding medical and nursing matters were the ANA, the NLN, and the AMA. The ANA was named by 35 percent (8) of the RNs, 13 percent (3) named the NLN, and 30 percent (7) named the AMA. The LPNs seemed to consider the NLN more important in this respect than the ANA. Only 17 percent (4) of the RNs were members of the ANA. Few of the nurses held any leadership positions in the community; the only positions noted were those of a social or religious nature; no nurse held a leadership role outside of the community. The faction that they felt would be most influential in promoting the acceptability of the PA concept was not the AMA or the public; it was the individual physicians by their expressed demand. This was in accord with the physicians' opinions on this issue.

Since the obstetrical PA would be working with the nurse, it is important to consider what effect the nurses felt the new worker would have upon the nurses' role. Only 5 percent (2) of the nurses felt the new job would be competitive with nursing and only one nurse felt that the new job might interfere with the present nurse-obstetrician working relationship; that is, only one felt that the nurse would have another "boss." This is in contrast to the physicians, some of whom felt these two effects might result from the use of the obstetrical PA. Forty-three percent (17) saw the new job as an opportunity for the nurse to expand her role in obstetrics by obtaining just a little more training. Forty percent (16) felt that the new job would take away from the nurse many of the "medical" functions which have fallen to her by default! These two findings were in agreement with the opinions of physicians.

As 88 percent of the physicians had expressed their satisfaction with their present obstetrical nurses, 75 percent of the obstetrical nurses were also satisfied with their present position. Only one nurse (a RN) did not feel that the physician gave her enough responsibility. However, 22 percent (5) of the RNs did not feel they were really "nursing;" this included 38 percent (3) of the eight office nurses.

Whereas the physicians had been fairly evenly divided in their opinions as to what effect the use of obstetrical PAs would have on the cost of obstetrical care, only 13 percent (5) of the nurses felt the PA would reduce the cost of care to the patient. The largest number of nurses (48 percent) felt that the use of the PA would increase the cost of care to the patient, and 35 percent (14) felt it would have no effect upon the cost. The reasons given for a possible reduction of the cost of obstetrical care were similar to those given by the doctors: (1) the PA's time would be less costly and therefore, patients without complications who use the PA's services would get care at less cost; and (2) since the doctors would spend less time with each patient they would be able to give care at less cost. Those nurses who felt the cost of obstetrical care would increase, strongly felt that the added cost of the PA's salary would be passed on to the patient in additional charges for obstetrical care. Three of the 18 nurses who felt it would increase costs felt that the patients would actually be receiving more care than they are presently and would be willing to pay more for it. The reasons given by those who felt the use of the PA would have no effect upon cost were: (1) more patients will be served by the obstetrician and his PA; therefore, the physician's net income will increase without increasing his cost to individual patients; and (2) the PA is very likely to become a hospital employee and, as such, would not affect the cost of obstetrical care to the patient.

Although 50 percent (4) of the obstetricians had emphasized the need for the "ideal" doctor to be professionally competent, 73 percent of the nurses stressed this trait as the "ideal" one. Fifty percent of the doctors had emphasized honesty with patients and ability to empathize with patients; only 20 percent of the nurses viewed this as the most important attribute for a good doctor to possess. Fifty-five percent (22) of the nurses felt the "ideal nurse" should be competent and efficient above all else while 20 percent (8) emphasized the need for the nurse to have a genuine concern for the patients' welfare; again, the doctors had split 50-50 on these traits for the "ideal" nurse. Sixty-three percent (25) of the nurses felt the "good patient" was one who faithfully carried out doctor's orders. Ten (25 percent) suggested that the "good patient" was one who reported health problems promptly.

The nurses saw two major advantages for the use of an obstetrical PA: (1) his use could provide more medical care to more people; and (2) since the PA would care for the needs of many of the patients without complications, his use would free the physician to spend more time with those needing his care more urgently. Twenty-three percent (9) of the nurses cited two additional advantages: (1) the obstetrical PA may be more readily available to the nurse and to the patient than the physician often is in an emergency situation; and (2) his use would free the nurse to spend more time in teaching and in meeting the psychosocial needs of women in pregnancy. The nurses noted few disadvantages that were likely to occur in employing PAs in obstetrics. Ten percent (4) feared the PA might become overconfident and carry out procedures without proper supervision. Only 7.5 percent (three nurses) feared a decrease in the closeness of the doctor-patient relationship or feared a loss of "prestige functions" by the nurse. The major potential disadvantage seen was the need to give sufficient lead time in initiating the use of the new worker; 30 percent (12) felt there must be sufficient time given to foster the faith and respect of the nurse and patient for the PA. In their view, a thorough understanding of the obstetrical PA's role must accompany his gradual introduction into the obstetrical field.

TASK ANALYSIS

Seventy-five percent of the obstetricians saw a need for and would use an obstetrical PA; 88 percent of the nurses saw a need for such a new health professional in obstetrics. From these findings, one could conclude that, at least in the one medium-sized southern city studied, there is a need for additional health professionals such as the PA in the obstetrical field. However, unless the potential job that needs to be fulfilled is well defined, one does not really know what the actual need is, or if the new worker will fill that need. A preliminary list of obstetrical office and hospital patient care tasks was compiled and the nurses and physicians were asked to indicate what tasks they felt would or would not be appropriate ones to delegate to an obstetrical PA; in addition, the nurses were asked: (1) what tasks they now perform in obstetrical nursing; (2) which tasks they feel they could perform now (without additional training) if delegated to them; and (3) which tasks they would be willing to do if they received additional training. (See Tables 6.4 and 6.5.)

Tables 6.4 and 6.5 indicate strong agreement between the nurses and physicians with regard to what tasks could be appropriately delegated to the PA. More than 50 percent of both doctors and nurses would delegate the following tasks to the obstetrical PA: pap smear, routine prenatal care, assisting with a Caesarean delivery, delivery of normal primipara, delivery of normal multipara, administration of intravenous therapy, administration of blood, management of routine postpartum care, postpartum hospital visits, follow-up postpartum home visits, and six-week postpartum check-ups. The physicians

TABLE 6.4

Opinions of the Obstetricians and the Obstetrical Office Nurses Regarding Office Patient Care Task Delegation

	Attitudes Toward Delegation[1]				
	A	B	C	D	E
Tasks	% (f)	% (f)	% (f)	% (f)	% (f)
INITIAL PHYSICAL ASSESSMENT					
Initial history and physical (excluding pelvic)	50 (4)	38 (3)	0 (0)	0 (0)	25 (2)
Initial pelvic examination	0 (0)	25 (2)	0 (0)	0 (0)	25 (2)
Pap smear	50 (4)	63 (5)	0 (0)	25 (2)	50 (4)
Pelvimetry, physical	13 (1)	63 (5)	0 (0)	25 (2)	38 (3)
Laboratory Tests					
Pregnancy tests	100 (8)	75 (6)	50 (4)	13 (1)	0 (0)
Complete blood count	88 (7)	38 (3)	0 (0)	0 (0)	38 (3)
Urinalysis	100 (8)	75 (6)	38 (3)	13 (1)	13 (1)
Blood typing	75 (6)	38 (3)	0 (0)	0 (0)	38 (3)
VDRL	75 (6)	38 (3)	0 (0)	0 (0)	38 (3)
Coombs test	75 (6)	38 (3)	0 (0)	0 (0)	38 (3)
PRENATAL CARE AND TREATMENT					
Routine prenatal care	88 (7)	88 (7)	13 (1)	25 (2)	25 (2)
Make emergency room visits	13 (1)	25 (2)	0 (0)	0 (0)	25 (2)
Take "on-call"	0 (0)	25 (2)	0 (0)	0 (0)	25 (2)
Primary treatment for pre-eclampsia	0 (0)	0 (0)	0 (0)	0 (0)	13 (1)
Follow-up treatment for pre-eclampsia	0 (0)	25 (2)	0 (0)	13 (1)	25 (2)
Primary treatment for eclampsia	0 (0)	0 (0)	0 (0)	0 (0)	13 (1)
Follow-up treatment for eclampsia	0 (0)	13 (1)	0 (0)	13 (1)	13 (1)
Follow-up postpartum home visits	88 (7)	75 (6)	0 (0)	0 (0)	38 (3)
Routine 6-week postpartum Checkup	50 (4)	75 (6)	0 (0)	0 (0)	38 (3)

[1]A = Obstetricians who favor task delegation to the obstetrical PA; N = 8.

B = Obstetrical office nurses who favor task delegation to the obstetrical PA; N = 8 (7 RNs and 1 LPN).

C = Tasks which the obstetrical office nurses are presently delegated; N = 8.

D = Tasks which the obstetrical office nurses feel they could do if so delegated, without any additional training; N = 8.

E = Tasks which the obstetrical office nurses feel they would be willing to do if they received additional training; N = 8.

Source: Compiled by the author.

TABLE 6.5

Opinions of the Obstetricians and the Obstetrical Hospital Nurses Regarding Hospital Patient Care Task Delegation

	Attitudes Toward Delegation[1]				
	A	B	C	D	E
Tasks	% (f)	% (f)	% (f)	% (f)	% (f)
LABOR AND DELIVERY TASKS					
Anesthesia Administration[2]					
General	25 (2)	31 (10)	0 (0)	0 (0)	22 (7)
Spinal	13 (1)	3 (1)	0 (0)	0 (0)	19 (6)
Saddle block	13 (1)	9 (3)	0 (0)	0 (0)	19 (6)
Pudendal	38 (3)	41 (13)	0 (0)	3 (1)	31 (10)
Paracervical	13 (1)	12 (4)	0 (0)	0 (0)	28 (9)
Assist with Caesarean delivery	75 (6)	63 (20)	0 (0)	3 (1)	41 (13)
Deliver normal primipara	50 (4)	75 (24)	0 (0)	9 (3)	31 (10)
Deliver normal multipara	75 (6)	78 (25)	3 (1)	16 (5)	28 (9)
Deliver multiple birth	0 (0)	37 (12)	0 (0)	12 (4)	19 (6)
Deliver breech birth	0 (0)	19 (6)	0 (0)	9 (3)	28 (9)
Administer intravenous therapy	88 (7)	91 (29)	25 (8)	9 (3)	22 (7)
Do venous cut-downs	38 (3)	25 (8)	0 (0)	3 (1)	22 (7)
Administer blood	75 (6)	78 (25)	22 (7)	9 (3)	19 (6)
Do exchange transfusion for newborn	0 (0)	3 (1)	0 (0)	0 (0)	19 (6)
Do intrauterine fetal transfusion	0 (0)	0 (0)	0 (0)	0 (0)	13 (4)
Do amniotic fluid evaluation	13 (1)	25 (8)	0 (0)	3 (1)	16 (5)
Use low outlet forceps	13 (1)	28 (9)	0 (0)	3 (1)	25 (8)
HOSPITAL POSTPARTUM CARE					
Manage routine postpartum care	88 (7)	84 (27)	19 (6)	9 (3)	19 (6)
Make postpartum hospital visits	75 (6)	97 (31)	0 (0)	6 (2)	28 (9)

[1] A = Obstetricians who favor task delegation to the obstetrical PA; N = 8.

B = Obstetrical hospital nurses who favor task delegation to the obstetrical PA; N = 32 (16 RNs and 16 LPNs). Nine of the LPNs work in the smaller of the two general hospitals where many of the obstetrical hospital tasks are, by necessity, done by LPNs; thus the experience with many obstetrical hospital tasks is very between the RNs and the LPNs.

C = Tasks which the obstetrical hospital nurses are presently delegated; N = 32.

D = Tasks which the obstetrical hospital nurses feel they could do if so delegated, without additional training; N = 32.

E = Tasks which the obstetrical hospital nurses feel they would be willing to do if they received additional training.

[2] Anesthesia is presently administered by nurse anesthetists under the direction of the attending obstetrician in the two local general hospitals.

Source: Compiled by the author.

FIGURE 6.1

Office Patient Care Tasks According to Present Delegation to Office Nurses and Opinion About Their Delegation to the Obstetrical Physician's Assistant

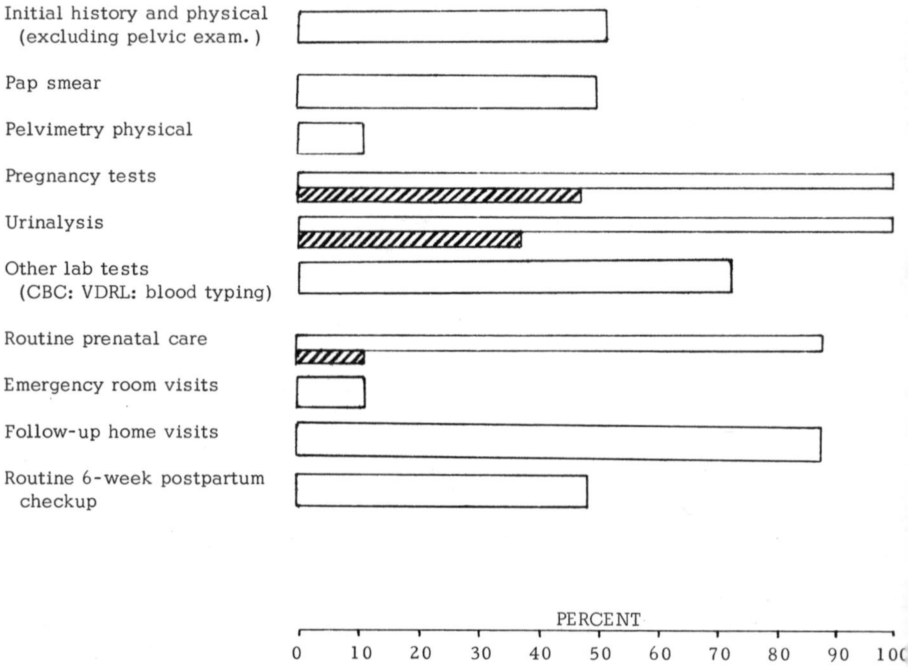

Obstetricians favor delegation to the obstetrical PA. N = 8.

Obstetrical office nurses are presently delegated this task by the physicians (as reported by the office nurses). N = 8.

Source: Compiled by the author.

FIGURE 6.2

Hospital Patient Care Tasks According to Present Delegation to Hospital Nurses and Opinion About Their Delegation to the Obstetrical Physician's Assistant

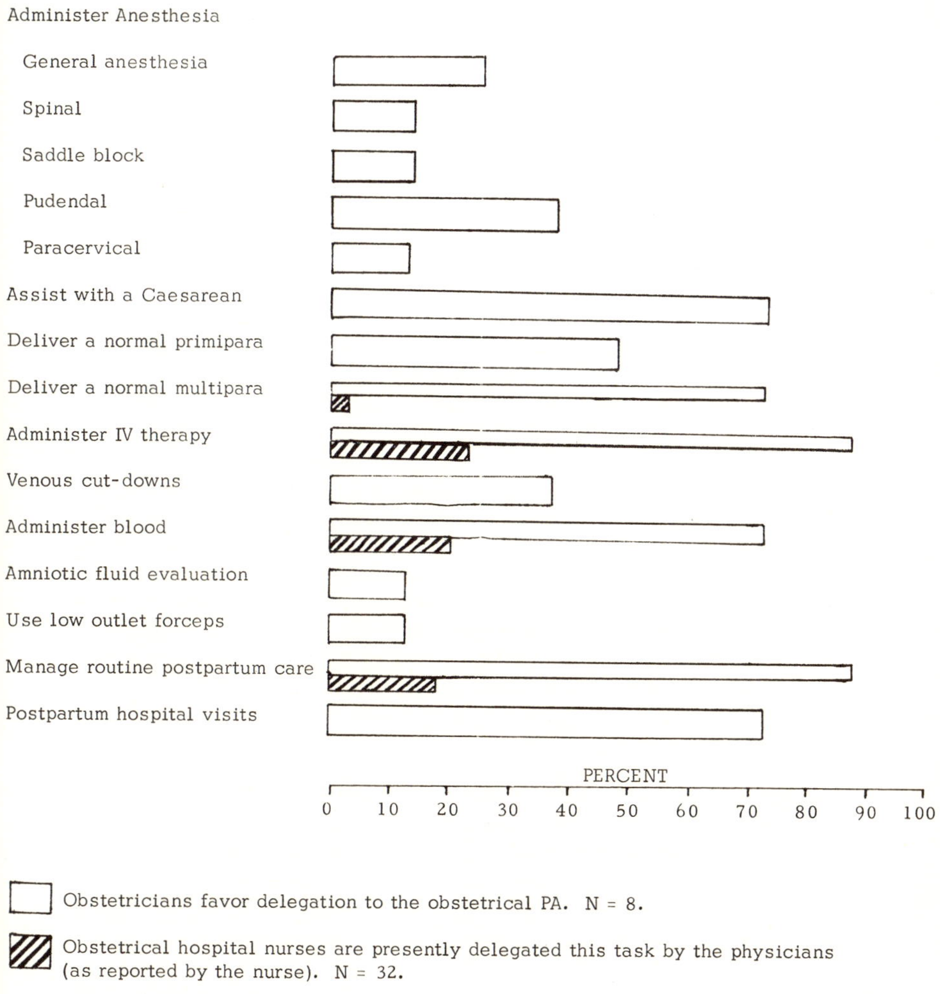

Source: Compiled by the author.

also felt that the initial history and physical examination (excluding the pelvic examination) and all laboratory tests could be delegated to the obstetrical PA. Only 38 percent (3) of the office nurses favored the former's delegation; the pregnancy test was the only laboratory test the nurses favored delegating to the PA. From remarks made by the nurses with regard to the delegation of laboratory tests, they apparently felt such tests would be "a waste of the PA's time;" these tasks could be performed (as they are today) by trained laboratory technicians. More than 50 percent of the nurses felt that physical pelvimetry could be carried out by the PA while only 13 percent (one) of the physicians felt this would be a proper delegation. Tables 6.4 and 6.5 further indicate that although the obstetrical nurses are presently delegated few "medical type" obstetrical tasks, few obstetrical nurses feel confident to assume these tasks without first receiving additional training. This finding related to the prior statement of job satisfaction by 75 percent of the nurses suggests that the obstetrical nurses are not being poorly utilized in their own (or in the physicians') estimation. However, that many of the obstetrical nurses were willing to assume more responsibility if they received further training, suggests that their value in obstetrics could be substantially enhanced.

Figures 6.1 and 6.2 visually compare those tasks the obstetricians feel could be appropriately delegated to a PA and what percentage of these tasks are presently delegated to their nurse assistants. By measuring the gap between "would delegate" and "presently delegated," one can begin to visualize the potential role which the obstetrical PA could fulfill and how useful his introduction into the field of obstetrics could be. By continuing this research one step farther, one could complete cost-benefit and cost-effectiveness analyses of these tasks and determine how valuable (in terms of both economic efficiency and noneconomic effectiveness) this new worker might be. (This last step was beyond the scope of the present study.)

POSSIBLE IMPLICATIONS AND SOME WORKING HYPOTHESES

The local study of the potential need for and acceptability of an obstetrical PA is unique in that it isolated all components of a segment of the medical community in a medium-sized city: obstetricians, obstetrical nurses, and obstetrical patients. As an exploratory examination of a health manpower problem, the analysis is suggestive of certain working hypotheses.

During the initial phases of this research in 1970, one prominent director of a PA training program cautioned the researcher that the selection of the obstetrical area as the focus for this aspect of the research might unduly bias the results against the introduction of a PA. His caution was twofold:

First, those physicians practicing in obstetrics are somewhat reluctant to introduce anyone other than a female into the practice setting. Second, there does exist a certain puritanistic attitude throughout society in relation to examining female patients.[4]

The researcher felt these two assertions were testable. Since the research was not limiting the concept of PA to males only, the first argument may not apply. However, the physician respondents did validate the assertion that they (the physicians) would favor a female for the role of obstetrical PA. With this in mind, it is important to note that neither the patients nor the nurses expressed any sex preference for the individuals chosen to fulfill the role of the PA. In fact, 20 percent (9) of the patients favored a male for the role while only 13 percent (6) favored a female. This finding certainly questions the validity of the second argument, if the opinions of the patients are to be considered. On the basis of these findings, one may consider a number of hypotheses.

Hypothesis No. 1: Although obstetricians may favor the female to become the obstetrical PA, the patients and the nurses would accept either sex in the role. Proven competency, not sex, will be the determining factor in promoting the acceptability of the PA.

The data suggested that the level of education and the term of a woman's pregnancy were factors to be considered in the introduction of an obstetrical PA.* From the study findings, the following hypotheses were constructed:

Hypothesis No. 2: Although education appears to not be clearly and systemically related to the degree of acceptance of the PA, it may be that acceptance of specific task delegation to the PA will be greatest in the least educated and in the most highly educated groups; acceptance will be least in the middle-range educated group.

Hypothesis No. 3: Women first introduced to the concept of the PA in their latter months of pregnancy tend to be less accepting both in principle and in specific task

---

*It will be remembered that the patient group was a relatively highly educated one; the least well educated were defined as those with a high school education or less; the middle-range educated were those with college and the highly educated were those with more than a 4-year college education.

delegation than those women who are introduced to the concept in their early months of pregnancy.

Hypothesis No. 3 is particularly relevant when drawing a sample; in order to present a true picture of attitudes toward an obstetrical PA, the same should be composed of equal numbers of patients in each term of pregnancy. (The study had 14 percent, 43 percent, and 43 percent of the patients in their first, second, and third trimester, respectively.)

The effect of the obstetrical PA upon the cost of obstetrical care is, and will undoubtedly continue to be, an important issue. The local physicians were undecided about what effect the obstetrical PA would have upon the cost of obstetrical care. The nurses suggested that costs would probably rise, whereas the patients stated they would be more accepting of the PA if his presence meant that the cost of care would be reduced. On the basis of the findings of this particular study then, the following working hypotheses were formulated:

> Hypothesis No. 4: If the use of a PA would mean a reduction in the cost of health care to the individual patient, the acceptability of his use by the patient will be enhanced.

> Hypothesis No. 5: Knowledge of the effect of the PA upon the cost of health care will not in itself be useful in predicting the attitude of the other health professionals toward the use of the PA.

The majority of the physicians, nurses, and patients in the study favored the recruitment of the RN for the new job of obstetrical PA. In addition, the patients favored the college graduate with a health-related major as a possible source for the obstetrical PA. The nurses also suggested this latter group as well as suggesting the use of ex-military medical corpsmen. The fact that the RN was already a familiar health worker who was accepted by the public and by the other health workers was given by all groups as the main reason for their selection. Relevant education and practical experience were also important in selecting a recruitment source.

> Hypothesis No. 6. PAs who are already RNs will most easily gain acceptance in their new role by physicians, patients, and other health professionals.

> Hypothesis No. 7. With demonstrated competency, college graduates with a health-related major and ex-military medical corpsmen will also prove acceptable as PAs.

There was considerable difficulty in delineating the nurses' role in obstetrics. The majority of physicians, nurses, and patients felt that there were definite roles for both the nurse and the PA to play in obstetrics. Eighty-eight percent of the doctors and 75 percent of the nurses were satisfied with the nurses' jobs in obstetrics. The physicians indicated that the jobs of nurse and PA may prove competitive and the PA may, in effect, become a second "boss" to the nurse. However, the nurses did not have these fears. They viewed the PA as a helpmate and as a possible career ladder for those nurses who wished to avail themselves of this new opportunity. The patients, although unclear with regard to the nurse's role in obstetrics, did not want the PA to replace the obstetrical nurse.

> Hypothesis No. 8. There is a need for both the nurse and the PA in obstetrics; however, there is a definite need to clearly delineate the respective roles of each, in order to better utilize and evaluate the contribution of each to the provision of optimum health care.

> Hypothesis No. 9. If the nurse understands the role of the PA, she will not view it as a threat to her own position, but will view it as a complementary career to her own and one which may provide her with a career ladder.

Knowledge of how the "ideal" is perceived is often helpful in identifying the type of worker required in a particular situation. Approximately 40 percent of the patients emphasized competency in the "ideal doctor," and 30 percent emphasized their need for the doctor to exhibit some concern for them as individuals. Fifty percent of the physicians emphasized concern for the patient as the most important attribute of a good nurse or doctor, and 50 percent emphasized competency for both. The nurses favored competency over concern in their evaluation of what makes a good doctor or nurse.

> Hypothesis No. 10. The good PA must have both competency and concern for his patients if he is to be acceptable to the majority of physicians, nurses, and patients.

There is considerable agreement among the physicians and nurses with regard to the resolution of any legal problems associated with the use of the PA. The respondents perceived that the doctrine of *respondeat superior* would cover many of the problems dealing with professional liability. Licensure was felt to act as a "policing" device. However, based upon the findings of the national surveys (Chapters 4 and 5), there is more to the legal issues than has been considered by the respondents in the local study. Since there is such a discrepancy between national and local findings with regard to the issue of licensure, it would appear that there is a need for more communication between the individual nurses and doctors and the professional organizations and educational programs who are studying these issues.

Both the nurses and the physicians maintained that neither the professional organizations nor the public would be the most important force in promoting the acceptability of the PA. They both felt that the individual physicians, by their expressed demand, would have the most powerful voices in instituting this manpower program. The local physicians were unaware of the AMA's position on the nurses' potential role as a PA. Although a majority of the RNs "agreed" with an ANA-NLN position on nurses and the PA, their agreement was based upon a misunderstanding of their professional organizations' positions; that is, although "agreeing" with the ANA-NLN position, they did not see the position as negating active support for the use of RNs as PAs. Thus, it appears that the constituencies of the professional organizations are sometimes neither aware of nor in agreement with their organizations' stated official positions.

> <u>Hypothesis No. 11</u>. When a professional organization is truly representative of its constituency, there will be receptive communication between all levels of the organization; that is, communication will be evidenced by the constituencies' knowledge and support of the organizations' official positions.

Both the physicians and the nurses saw more advantages than disadvantages for the use of the PA. They both agreed upon the major advantages:

> <u>Hypothesis No. 12</u>. An advantage that health professionals will perceive resulting from the use of the PA is that the PA will free the physician of much routine care, so that the seriously ill will receive more care.

> <u>Hypothesis No. 13</u>. An advantage that health professionals will perceive resulting from the use of the PA is that the physician will be able to give more care to more patients.

The patient group also perceived the advantages that were suggested by the physicians and by the nurses. In addition, they saw the PA as someone who would be able to take the time to talk with them about their pregnancy and really listen to their problems. A potential disadvantage was the fear that the doctor may increase his patient load so that the routine patient would rarely see the doctor unless a serious problem arose. It was noted that none of the most highly educated group were concerned about receiving inferior care if they used the services of the PA, while this fear was most often cited by those with the least amount of education. Since income is often equated with education, this latter group could also be considered the potentially low income group; thus, it appears inadvisable that

PAs be programmed to serve primarily low income groups. In order to allay this fear of inferior care by those with the least education, it is suggested that:

> Hypothesis No. 14. In order that the PA most successfully contribute to the development of a better health care delivery system, his services must be made available to and used by all segments (income and education groups) of the society.

In order to promote the successful adoption of the PA, the nurses perceived a need to provide sufficient lead time in initiating the use of the new health professional. The PA is needed and will be used; however, the manner in which he is introduced into the health field is important.

> Hypothesis No. 15. The introduction of the PA into the health field will be most successful if his role is well defined, his introduction is gradual, and his position as a member of the health team is stressed.

NOTES

1. American Medical Association's Committee on Nursing, "Medicine and Nursing in the 1970s: A Position Statement," Journal of the American Medical Association 213, no. 11 (September 1970): 1881-1883.
2. Ibid.
3. Eileen M. Jacobi, "Officially Speaking...," RN 33, no. 10 (October 1970): 57, 82, 84; Margaret E. Walsh, "Officially Speaking ...," RN 33, no. 10 (October 1970): 84, 86, 88.
4. Letter from D. Robert Howard, M. D., Director, Physician's Assistant Program, Duke University Medical Center, Durham, North Carolina, January 11, 1971.

CHAPTER

7

CONCLUDING REMARKS AND IMPLICATIONS

The physician's assistant grew out of a perceived need—the need to provide health care services of better quality and greater quantity to more people. This need and service orientation should not be lost sight of in debating the advantages and disadvantages of the innovation. This book has dealt extensively with many of the basic issues that must of necessity be resolved if the PA is to emerge as a viable contributor to health service delivery. Issues such as role definition, legal accommodation, cost factors, recruitment problems, acceptability by other providers and by the public are all of vital importance. However, they are all only reduced to academic significance if the end result is not the desired one—improved accessibility to high quality health care.

Advocates of change are often put in an uncomfortable position. They must sell a change to the existing system. In their desire to see their innovation accepted, they run the risk of being coopted by that system. To fit the PA into the system is not enough. The introduction of the PA should be viewed as an opportunity to revitalize the system—to subject it to the scrutiny that is required. The conflict that is generated by change is healthy. True, conflict can be divisive—it can degenerate into destructive self-aggrandizement by parties with vested interests in maintaining the status quo. However, it is the task of the wary change agent to prevent such degeneration. One means of doing so is to subject planned change to the examination it deserves. Theory can suggest potential problems upon which data can then be systematically gathered and analyzed. The final justification for such data, however, is in its application. Thus, the researcher disseminates his findings in the hopes or providing direction for the change agents—and of elevating the level at which conflict takes place.

The introduction of the PA has generated conflict. It has forced those who were comfortable with the status quo to re-examine their positions. The two major health professional associations have responded to a long felt need for more collaborative planning. That the PA is demanding inclusion in such collaborative efforts will open the system to further change than might otherwise have resulted from such efforts. The introduction of the PA has been a major force in encouraging the nursing profession to re-examine its role, acknowledge its inadequacies—and assert its right (and responsibility) to play a greater role in health care delivery. Rigidities in the system, such as licensure, have become more apparent and are now being subjected to study. The issue is not only whether the PA as a new health provider is to be licensed, but whether the whole system of licensure is in itself archaic—unable to meet the needs of a dynamic health system where-ever greater demands are being placed on providers. The issue of reimbursement is now a focal point of debate. It is not simply whether the PA or NP are to be eligible for third-party reimbursement, but whether reimbursement policies can be used to effectively restructure the system in order to provide new types of services in new ways (such as different combinations of health manpower, technology, and organizational arrangements).

We too often tend to see innovations in isolation: a new means of financing health care (for example, national health insurance), a new type of health provider (for example, the PA), a new mode of organizing health services (for example, health maintenance organizations). Obviously, the ramifications of a single change are many. The effect of simultaneously related change is overwhelming—and invigorating.

One could enumerate an extensive list of policy implications emanating from this study. Several will be mentioned here but, in keeping with the author's intentions, it is left to the reader to derive his own implications. Exploratory studies do not dictate answers—they provide direction.

Opportunities for career mobility in the health fields have, to date, been inadequate. The new PA profession affords a career ladder to lower level health workers (medical corpsmen, for example) and should, in turn, provide a foundation for further advancement (for example, advanced placement in medical school). In order to facilitate mobility, career ladders (lateral and vertical) should be encouraged throughout the health area. A core health science curriculum could be developed to provide the necessary preparation for such mobility. A logical extension of this approach would be the establishment of a continuum of health science degrees perhaps along the lines suggested recently by Harry I. Greenfield; that is, doctor of medicine (M. D.), master of science in medicine, bachelor of science in medicine (B. S. in Med.), and associate of arts in medicine.[1] Others have also proposed the development of multiple levels of health and medical care practitioners.[2] This approach has been used with considerable success in other countries.*

The PA's role as a member of the health care team should be stressed. The team should be a fluid one—the leadership and composition of which changes as dictated by the needs of the patient. This is similar to an approach suggested by Edmund Pellegrino.[3] The development of a core health science curriculum should reinforce this concept—in the early stages of a prospective health provider's career before professional lines are solidified. Multidisciplinary clinical teams should be introduced early in professional training as well, in order to promote mutual respect for the unique contributions of each of the many health care providers.

As the PA will (or should) be a force for change within the system, so changes in the system will affect the development of the PA. The widespread adoption of HMOs will obviously affect the use of PAs. More and more PAs would be employed by these health care organizations and utilized either within a central facility or deployed in satellite units of a regional health care complex. In such situations, the one-to-one relationship between a PA and his physician-employer may no longer exist. Ever greater emphasis would be placed on providing preventive care and health education as well as a need for an increasing degree of sophistication in the use of diagnostic facilities. The introduction of national health insurance would not only affect the numbers of health providers needed to meet the anticipated increased demands, but will affect the types of services which are to be reimbursed; thus the PA may find his role significantly altered. The educators of PAs must be aware of and anticipate these changes in order to prepare the PA to readily adapt to these new responsibilities.

The PA must not be the purveyor of second-class medicine. His services must be made available to all segments of society. Although his services will be needed in urban ghettos and rural areas, his use must not be limited to such areas. At the same time, he should not become an instrument of exploitation, being employed predominately in lucrative urban practices. The maldistribution of physicians that is present in the United States today (and compounds any numerical shortage which may exist) should not be replicated by an equivalent maldistribution of PAs. In order to minimize such an occurrence,

---

*Those who advocate the use of multiple levels of medical care practitioners should be cognizant, however, of some of the difficulties which may result. For example, the British health system is organized along these lines; many valuable insights could be gained by a perusal of the recent critique of medical education in Great Britain. See Royal Commission on Medical Education 1965-68: Report (London, England: Her Majesty's Stationery Office, 1969).

adequate provision must be made to accommodate the use of PAs in areas or settings physically distant from their employers.

With the cost of medical care continuously rising, an increase in the numbers of highly trained physicians may well accelerate the rising costs to intolerable heights. Even if the costs did not skyrocket, there is no assurance that an increase in the numbers of highly educated physicians will solve the health manpower shortage. An increase in physicians will not improve the inequitable distribution of physicians that exists in the United States today.

What is the solution to our health manpower shortage? Obviously, there is no single answer. The physician shortage cannot, however, be simplistically resolved by increasing the supply of physicians. Rather, one must develop ways to utilize our present health manpower more efficiently and devise new methods of fulfilling manpower requirements. In the past, physician support personnel have been generally of the modest education, low salary variety. The degree of independent functioning of these types of personnel has been (and is) almost nonexistent. Perhaps it is time that we gave our physicians a genuine assistant—one who is able to function with a substantial degree of autonomy. Only in this way can a taut supply of well-educated (and well paid) physicians continue to provide quality health care for our increasing population. By increasing the ability of each physician to treat more patients, the use of PAs should reduce the total number of physicians needed.

The PA was introduced as a means to increase the productivity of existing health professionals. That he can do this has been fairly well substantiated. However, what was not fully anticipated was his development into a health professional in his own right. Albeit he is still legally dependent on the physician, his own areas of expertise are constantly growing. The PA of even a few years ago was first and foremost a technician; today, the PA is considered by many to be a new primary health care professional.

NOTES

1. Michael M. Dasco, "Training of Allied Health Professionals and Physicians' Assistants," Bulletin of the New York Academy of Medicine 46, no. 12 (December 1970): 1109-1110.

2. Henry K. Silver, "A New Primary-Care Medical Practitioner," American Journal of Diseases of Children 126 (September 1973), pp. 324-327; E. F. Rosinski, "Education and the Role of the Physician," Journal of the American Medical Association 222 (1972), pp. 473-475; S. Proger, "The Education of Different Types of Physicians for Different Types of Health Care," Pharos 35 (1972), pp. 53-66.

3. Edmund Pellegrino, The Changing Matrix of Clinical Decision-Making (Ann Arbor: University of Michigan Institute for Social Research, 1970), Chapters IV, V, cited in Alfred M. Sadler, Blair L. Sadler, and Ann A. Bliss, The Physician's Assistant: Today and Tomorrow (New Haven: Yale University Press, 1972), pp. 134-135.

APPENDIX A

1970 NATIONAL SURVEY QUESTIONNAIRE FOR PA PROGRAMS

The following questions were included in a letter sent to 33 operative and 10 planned PA training programs in the United States:

1. How does your program define the term "physician's assistant"?

2. What "type" (specialty orientation) of physician's assistant do you educate (or anticipate educating) in your program?

3. How did you develop the job description for your type of physician's assistant? (I would appreciate copies of any job descriptions which you have developed.)

4. What do you consider to be the proper recruitment source? Why?

5. What variables have you found which may be related to the acceptability (or rejection) of the physician's assistant by existing medical and paramedical personnel?

6. What factors do you feel will be the most important in promoting the acceptability of this new allied health professional?

7. a. By what means do you feel the legal question surrounding the use of "medical judgement" by a physician's assistant will (or should) be resolved?

   b. How do you feel it should be resolved?

8. How do you view the question of licensure for the physician's assistant? Why?

9. In what types of positions have your graduates been placed? Do you have any knowledge of the acceptability of your graduates in their new positions by the professionals, paraprofessionals, and client populations with whom they work? What appear to be your graduates' positive and negative characteristics?

10. Did you administer any survey of need for the physician's assistant in your area before instituting the program? (I would very much appreciate your sending copies of any questionnaires used in the study and any results you may have completed, if it is possible for you to do so.)

11. Did you survey the anticipated acceptability of the physician's assistant in your area before initiating your program? (Any questionnaires and results of these studies would be extremely helpful.)

APPENDIX B

1973 NATIONAL SURVEY QUESTIONNAIRE FOR PA PROGRAMS

(1) MANY NEW PROGRAMS ARE BEING DEVELOPED WITH THE OVERALL GOAL OF INCREASING BOTH THE EFFICIENCY AND EQUITY OF HEALTH CARE DELIVERY. THE PHYSICIAN'S ASSISTANT (PA) AND THE NURSE PRACTITIONER (NP) ARE GENERIC TERMS USED TO DESCRIBE TWO OF THESE NEW MEDICAL-ALLIED HEALTH PROFESSIONALS.

(A) PLEASE INDICATE WHICH TYPE OF MEDICAL-ALLIED HEALTH PROFESSIONAL YOU EDUCATE IN YOUR PROGRAM (NOTING A SPECIALTY ORIENTATION WHERE APPROPRIATE).

____

(B) HOW DOES YOUR PROGRAM DEFINE THE TERM "PHYSICIAN'S ASSISTANT" OR "NURSE PRACTITIONER" (WHICHEVER IS APPLICABLE)?

____
____
____
____
____
____

(C) HOWEVER YOU DEFINED THE TERM PA OR NP, YOU WILL PROBABLY HAVE INCLUDED SOME EQUIVALENT OF THE PHRASE ". . . WORK WITH AND UNDER THE SUPERVISION OF A PHYSICIAN." OF THE FOLLOWING INTERPRETATIONS OF THIS PHRASE, <u>WHICH ONES</u> BEST REPRESENT YOUR PROGRAM'S USE OF THE PHRASE? (YOU WILL PROBABLY WANT TO SELECT SEVERAL.)

____ the apostrophe in "physician's assistant" makes the phrase singularly possessive and not plurally possessive; i.e., the PA or NP must be employed by a single physician.

____ the apostrophe in "physician's assistant" is misplaced; it should be physicians' assistant; i.e., the PA or NP can be employed by a group of physicians or function under the auspices of a hospital's medical staff.

____ the PA or NP must always work in close proximity of his employer; i.e., he must always work in the same office as his physician-employer in order to be "under his supervision."

____ the PA or NP could work in a setting physically removed from that of his employer as long as effective lines of communication are available at all times; for example, telephone, two-way video transmissions, etc. . . .

____ all procedures performed by the PA or NP must be able to be directly reviewed by his physician-employer; sporadic review is not sufficient.

____ It is sufficient that procedures performed by a NP or PA be subject to "review as needed;" to require direct review of all procedures will unduly hamper the use of these new workers.

____ Other (please be specific) ______________________________
____
____
____

(D) WE HAVE CHOSEN TO CLASSIFY BOTH THE PA AND THE NP AS 'HEALTH PROFESSIONALS' WHO ARE 'ALLIED WITH THE MEDICAL PROFESSION.'

(1) HOW WOULD YOU CLASSIFY THE GRADUATES OF YOUR PROGRAM?

____ health professionals
____ allied health professionals
____ medical-allied health professionals
____ Other (please be specific) ______________________

(2) WHY HAVE YOU CHOSEN THIS CLASSIFICATION? SHORT CONCISE PHRASES ARE SUFFICIENT.

(2) THE TASK OF DEVELOPING AN ACCEPTABLE JOB DESCRIPTION FOR A NEW HEALTH WORKER IS A DIFFICULT ONE. DUE TO THE DIVERSE NATURE OF MANY OF THE PROGRAMS EDUCATING PAs OR NPs, MANY DIFFERENT APPROACHES HAVE BEEN UTILIZED.

(A) PLEASE SELECT FROM THE APPROACH(ES) LISTED BELOW THE ONE(S) WHICH MUST CLOSELY APPROXIMATES THE MANNER

IN WHICH YOUR PROGRAM INITIALLY DEVELOPED THE NECESSARY JOB DESCRIPTION. YOU MAY HAVE USED A COMBINATION OF APPROACHES; IF SO, PLEASE INDICATE YOUR PRIMARY APPROACH BY THE NUMBER 1 AND MERELY CHECK SUPPLEMENTARY ONES.

____ a) adopted guidelines for a Type 'A', 'B', or 'C' physician's assistant as defined by the 1970 National Academy of Sciences' report on the PA. Please indicate if you chose Type A ____, Type B ____, Type C ____)

____ b) adopted guidelines developed by a Joint Committee of the ANA and the relevant medical specialty professional organizations; for example, the American Academy of Pediatrics or the American College of Obstetrics and Gynecology.

____ c) adopted guidelines established by the AMA's Council on Medical Education in collaboration with the relevant professional organization of potential physician-employers; for example, the American Urological Association or the American Academy of Orthopaedic Surgeons.

____ d) adopted guidelines only after conducting a task analysis (or reviewing the results of previous studies in the relevant functional area) of the specialist or general practitioner with whom the PA or NP is to work; the task analysis highlighted the tasks which could be assumed by the PA or NP so that the educational program could focus on these tasks when developing a job description.

____ e) examined the health needs of a particular target population and developed a job description which would meet these potential patients' needs.

____ f) by survey, it was determined which tasks performed by a PA or NP would be acceptable to the patient and then these tasks were incorporated into a job description.

____ g) utilized the skills of an interdisciplinary advisory committee (including representatives from relevant academic departments, professional associations, hospitals, etc. ...) to develop broad categories of activities which a PA or NP could be expected to assume; these broad categories were then subjected to further refinement depending upon the specialty orientation of the PAs or NPs to be trained and/or the setting in which the individual would be expected to function.

____ h) a general skeletal job description was initially developed; students were studied as they proceeded through the program to determine how much, how fast, and how well they could learn and understand the necessary medical skills and techniques; gradually a more specific job description was formulated.

____ i) did not develop a specific job description; the program offered the PA or NP a generalist core curriculum and expected the individual student, with his specific physician-employer, to develop a more explicit job description once employed; this might involve additional on-the-job training.

____ j) Other (please be specific) ____________________________

____

____

____

____

(B) HAVING GAINED EXPERIENCE WITH THE PROGRAM, WOULD YOU TODAY HAVE SELECTED THE SAME APPROACH TO FORMULATING A JOB DESCRIPTION WHICH YOUR PROGRAM INITIALLY SELECTED?

____ Yes ____ No

____ IF NO, WHICH OF THE ABOVE APPROACHES WOULD YOU NOW USE TO FORMULATE A JOB DESCRIPTION FOR THE PA OR NP? PLEASE INDICATE THE LETTER OF THE APPROACH YOU WOULD NOW SELECT.

(3) THERE HAS BEEN SOME CONTROVERSY CONCERNING 'APPROPRIATE' RECRUITMENT SOURCES FOR A PHYSICIAN'S ASSISTANT.

(A) IF YOUR PROGRAM EDUCATES PAs, PLEASE INDICATE WHICH RECRUITMENT SOURCES YOUR PROGRAM NOW PREFERS; PLEASE RANK ORDER YOUR CHOICES USING THE RATING SCALE BELOW.

IF YOUR PROGRAM EDUCATES NPs, PLEASE INDICATE WHICH RECUITMENT SOURCES YOUR PROGRAM FEELS SHOULD BE RECRUITED FOR THE ROLE OF THE PA; PLEASE RANK ORDER YOUR CHOICES USING THE RATING SCALE BELOW.

1 = first preference
2 = second preference
3 = third preference
4 = fourth preference

____ college graduate, with a health-related major other than pre-med

____ college graduate with a pre-med major who is not accepted into medical school and/or decides not to attend medical school

____ college graduate, with a non-health-related major

____ registered nurse with a baccalaureate degree in nursing

____ registered nurse with a diploma or associate degree

____ practical nurse

____ allied health paraprofessionals (inhalation therapists, medical technicians, etc.)

____ discharged independent-duty medical corpsman

____ discharged medical corpsmen

____ high school graduate

____ Other (please be specific) ______________________________
____

(B) WITH REGARD TO YOUR FIRST PREFERENCE, WHY DO YOU FEEL THIS TYPE OF PERSON WOULD BE THE MOST APPROPRIATE TO RECRUIT FOR THE ROLE OF THE PHYSICIAN'S ASSISTANT? PLEASE RANK ORDER THE THREE MOST IMPORTANT REASONS FOR YOUR SELECTION OF THESE INDIVIDUALS ACCORDING TO THE FOLLOWING SCALE:

1 = most important reason
2 = second most important reason
3 = third most important reason

____ substantial potential supply available which is presently ill-utilized or not utilized at all by the health professions

____ highest degree of general education; thus greater potential to function at a high level in the new role with comparatively little additional preparation

____ highest degree of health-related education which would provide a good foundation for further advancement in the health field

____ more willing to train for, and function well in a dependent occupation

____ more willing and able to assume a role of increasing responsibility which will require a substantial degree of independent judgment

____ Other (please be specific) ______________________________
____
____

(4) SOME PHYSICIAN'S ASSISTANT PROGRAMS SEEM TO FAVOR THE RECRUITMENT OF ONE SEX OVER THE OTHER FOR THE PA ROLE. NURSE PRACTITIONER PROGRAMS BY DEFINITION RECRUIT NURSES; NURSING IS PREDOMINANTLY A FEMALE CAREER; THEREFORE, NP PROGRAMS PRIMARILY RECRUIT FEMALES.

THIS QUESTION RELATES SPECIFICALLY TO THE SUITABILITY OF ONE SEX VIS-A-VIS THE OTHER SEX FOR A CAREER AS A PA OR A NP.

(A) WHICH SEX DOES YOUR PROGRAM FEEL SHOULD BE RECRUITED FOR A CAREER AS A PA? (BOTH PA AND NP PROGRAMS SHOULD ANSWER THIS QUESTION.)

____ predominantly males ____ predominantly females
____ either

(B) WHICH SEX DOES YOUR PROGRAM FEEL SHOULD BE RECRUITED FOR A CAREER AS A NP? (BOTH PA AND NP PROGRAMS SHOULD ANSWER THIS QUESTION.)

____ predominantly males ____ predominantly females
____ either

(C) IF YOUR PROGRAM FAVORS MALES FOR THE ROLE OF THE PA AND/OR THE NP, PLEASE RANK ORDER THE TWO MOST IMPORTANT REASONS FOR SUCH SELECTION ACCORDING TO THE FOLLOWING SCALE:

1 = most important
2 = second most important

____ if the PA and/or NP roles were to be identified as acceptable male occupations, more males would be willing to pursue these careers; currently males are lost to many non-physician health professions due to the relatively low status and poor pay too often associated with predominantly female careers.

____ males are more geographically stable than females thus providing continuity to the health manpower supply in an area of need.

____ males are less restricted by home and family responsibilities and are therefore able to provide more dependable service as well as keep more flexible hours than females would be able to provide.

____ the male physician will be more willing to develop a truly collaborative relationship with a male PA or NP than he would with their female counterparts.

____ Other (please be specific) ______________________________
____
____
____

(D) IF YOUR PROGRAM FAVORS FEMALES FOR THE ROLE OF PA AND/OR THE NP, PLEASE RANK ORDER THE THREE MOST IMPORTANT REASONS FOR YOUR SELECTION ACCORDING TO THE FOLLOWING SCALE:

1 = most important
2 = second most important
3 = third most important

____ females are more readily accepted by patients than males to fulfill a non-physician role which involves direct patient care.

____ females are more empathetic and are needed as PAs or NPs to interject more personal concern into health care delivery.

____ physicians will more readily accept a female PA or NP (particularly if she has a nursing background) than they would be willing to accept a male PA or NP.

____ females are more willing to function in a physician-dependent role.

____ there will be less competition between a physician (still a predominantly male role in our society) and a female PA or NP thus promoting more cooperation and facilitating better health care delivery.

____ Other (please be specific) ______________________________
____
____
____

(E) IF YOUR PROGRAM FEELS THAT EITHER SEX WOULD FUNCTION EQUALLY WELL IN A PA AND/OR NP ROLE, PLEASE SUMMARIZE REASONS FOR YOUR SELECTION.

(5) REGISTERED NURSES ARE BEING RECRUITED BY PHYSICIAN'S ASSISTANT PROGRAMS.

(A) DOES YOUR PROGRAM FAVOR THE RECRUITMENT OF RNs INTO PHYSICIAN'S ASSISTANT PROGRAMS?

____ Yes ____ No

IF YES, COMPLETE (B), SKIP (C), AND GO TO (D) AND REST OF QUESTION (5).

IF NO, SKIP (B), AND GO TO (C) AND REST OF QUESTION (5).

(B) IF YOUR PROGRAM FAVORS THE RECRUITMENT OF REGISTERED NURSES AS PHYSICIAN'S ASSISTANTS, PLEASE RANK ORDER THE TWO MOST IMPORTANT REASONS FOR YOUR POSITION ACCORDING TO THE FOLLOWING SCALE:

1 = most important
2 = second most important

____ Nurses are ill-utilized; most of the tasks a nurse performs are routine and/or administrative in nature. A nurse practicing as a physician's assistant may find more opportunities to use her many skills (gained from both her nursing and her PA education) than she can presently find in her nursing practice.

____ The goal of all health professionals is to provide the best health care possible to their patients; if a nurse can broaden her skills by becoming a PA and thus provide better care to her patients, she should be encouraged to do so. Whether she is called a nurse, a NP or a PA is irrelevant.

____ There should be more upward and/or lateral mobility in the health professions with experience as well as formal education providing a basis for advancement; a nurse becoming a PA is an example of lateral mobility at the very least and might possibly be considered an example of upward career mobility.

____ There is a high degree of incongruity between nursing education and nursing practice; nursing education emphasizes intelligence, judgment, imagination, and empathy while nursing practice too often stresses efficiency, routinization, unquestioning obedience to 'doctor's orders'; playing the 'doctor–nurse game'; etc... This leads to dissatisfaction with the nurses' role and fosters early 'retirement'. The PA role, with its emphasis on the use of independent judgment and the development of a collaborative relationship with a physician-employer, might keep many nurses active and interested in providing health care.

____ Other (please be specific) ________________________________

____

____

____

(C) IF YOUR PROGRAM DOES NOT FAVOR THE RECRUITMENT OF REGISTERED NURSES AS PAs, PLEASE RANK ORDER THE THREE MOST IMPORTANT REASONS FOR YOUR POSITION ACCORDING TO THE FOLLOWING SCALE:

1 = most important
2 = second most important
3 = third most important

____ There is a shortage of working nurses in the U.S. today; if nurses are enticed into PA programs, this shortage of working nurses will become even more acute.

____ Nursing schools and colleges are for the education of nurses and not for the education of assistants to the physician; if PA programs recruit nurses for careers as PAs, nursing schools will have, in essence, provided some of the education for the PA.

____ Nurse practitioner programs build on nursing skills; they understand the important unique role nursing contributes to patient care; if RNs wish to expand their skills, they should be encouraged to enter NP programs and NOT encouraged to enter PA programs.

____ There should be a clear delineation of functions among the many health professionals; this is particularly important with regard to the nursing profession and the PA profession; if a nurse seeks further education as a PA, this would tend to blur the distinctions between the two careers.

____ Nurses who become PAs are not expanding their role; they are changing it! Those who encourage nurses to become PAs are encouraging nurses to leave nursing!

____ The use of a licensed RN, with a graduate certificate from a PA program, may lead to unforeseen legal difficulties; a nurse is licensed to practice nursing and is not licensed to function as a PA.

____ Other (please be specific) ______________________________
____
____
____

(D) WHAT DOES YOUR PROGRAM FEEL ARE THE ESSENTIAL DIFFERENCES BETWEEN THE ROLE OF THE 'TRADITIONAL REGISTERED NURSE' AND THE ROLE WHICH IS TO BE ASSUMED BY THE PHYSICIAN'S ASSISTANT? PLEASE INCLUDE EXAMPLES OF SPECIFIC TASKS WHICH YOU SEEM APPROPRIATE FOR THE PA BUT WHICH ARE NOT GENERALLY APPROPRIATE FOR THE TRADITIONAL REGISTERED NURSE.

(E) WHAT DOES YOUR PROGRAM FEEL ARE THE ESSENTIAL DIFFERENCES BETWEEN THE ROLE OF THE 'TRADITIONAL REGISTERED NURSE' AND THE ROLE WHICH IS TO BE ASSUMED BY THE NURSE PRACTITIONER? PLEASE INCLUDE EXAMPLES OF SPECIFIC TASKS WHICH YOU DEEM APPROPRIATE FOR THE NP BUT WHICH ARE NOT GENERALLY APPROPRIATE FOR THE TRADITIONAL REGISTERED NURSE.

(F) WHAT DOES YOUR PROGRAM FEEL ARE THE ESSENTIAL DIFFERENCES BETWEEN THE ROLE OF THE NURSE PRACTITIONER AND THE ROLE WHICH IS TO BE ASSUMED BY THE PHYSICIAN'S ASSISTANT? PLEASE INCLUDE EXAMPLES OF SPECIFIC TASKS WHICH YOU DEEM APPROPRIATE FOR THE PA BUT WHICH WOULD PROBABLY NOT BE CONSIDERED APPROPRIATE FOR THE NP. IN ADDITION, WHICH WOULD BE APPROPRIATE FOR THE NP BUT NOT FOR THE PA?

(G) SOME ASSERT THAT THE PA ROLE OFFERS AN UPWARD CAREER LADDER FOR THE NURSE. DO YOU AGREE OR DISAGREE WITH THIS ASSERTION? WHY?

____ Agree ____ Disagree

WHY? ____

____

____

____

(6) REGARDLESS OF ONE'S APPROVAL AND/OR DISAPPROVAL OF THE RECRUITMENT OF REGISTERED NURSES INTO PA AND/OR NP PROGRAMS, THE NURSE (FUNCTIONING AS A PA OR NP) IS FULFILLING A HEALTH CARE ROLE SOMEWHAT DIFFERENT FROM THAT WHICH IS PRESENTLY ASSUMED BY RNs. RNs ARE BEING ASKED TO FULFILL THESE ROLES—AND THEY ARE SHOWING THEIR WILLINGNESS TO DO SO BY ENTERING BOTH PA AND NP PROGRAMS.

(A) BASED ON YOUR PROGRAM'S EXPERIENCES, WHY DO YOU THINK REGISTERED NURSES ARE BEING ASKED TO PURSUE CAREERS AS PAs AND NPs? PLEASE RANK ORDER THE FOUR MOST IMPORTANT REASONS FOR YOUR POSITION ACCORDING TO THE FOLLOWING SCALE:

1 = most important
2 = second most important
3 = third most important
4 = fourth most important

____ utilizing nurses as PAs and NPs will promote general public acceptance of these new health professionals since the RN is already an accepted health care provider.

____ traditionally the RN and the physician have worked well together; therefore, the use of the RN in an expanded role (as PA or NP) will receive strong medical support and acceptance.

____ although the RN and the physician have worked well together in the past, their relationship has not always been as co-professionals; if the RN becomes a NP or PA, she will more readily be able to promote a collaborative relationship between medicine and nursing.

____ licensure problems would be minimal if an existing health professional, with additional education, assumed these new roles; most registered nurse practice acts are sufficiently permissive to allow the nurse to function in these expanded roles.

____ representing the largest pool (including both active and inactive nurses) of existing health workers, it was to be expected that innovative programs in health manpower would view RNs as likely candidates for their programs.

____ RNs who are recruited as PAs or NPs will be primarily those nurses who are currently inactive; these nurses will be enticed out of 'retirement' by the increased responsibility and increased remuneration which these new careers offer; therefore, recruiting nurses for expanded roles as PAs or NPs will not deplete the supply of practicing 'traditional registered nurses.'

____ Other (please be specific) ______________________________

____

____

____

(B) BASED ON YOUR PROGRAM'S GENERAL EXPERIENCE IN THE HEALTH MANPOWER AREA, <u>WHY DO YOU THINK MANY NURSES ARE WILLING TO PURSUE CAREERS AS PAs AND NPs</u>? PLEASE RANK ORDER THE THREE MOST IMPORTANT REASONS FOR YOUR POSITION ACCORDING TO THE FOLLOWING SCALE:

1 = most important
2 = second most important
3 = third most important

____ as a PA or NP, the RN feels she would receive greater remuneration for her services than her traditional nursing career can now offer her.

____ as a PA or NP, the RN feels she will be able to assume a greater degree of responsibility for patient care than she is presently able to do in her traditional nursing practice.

____ promotions in nursing too often involve movement away from direct patient care; the RN feels that the PA or NP career would mean advancement and yet still enable her to provide direct patient care.

____ RNs are beginning to view both PA and NP programs as offering them sorely needed career ladders through which nurses wishing to build upon and expand their skills may do so with comparatively little additional education; this is particularly true for the diploma nurse who finds little academic credit is given her hospital-based education by collegiate nursing programs.

____ RNs desire a more collaborative or co-professional relationship between themselves and physicians; they are beginning to view the emerging NP and PA programs as potentially offering them this opportunity which their traditional nursing practice has denied to them.

____ Other (please be specific) __________________________

____

____

____

(C) IN YOUR BEST ESTIMATION, <u>NURSE-RECRUITS FOR PHYSICIAN'S ASSISTANT PROGRAMS ARE PRIMARILY</u> WHICH OF THE FOLLOWING TYPES; PLEASE CHECK JUST ONE RESPONSE.

____ disillusioned with nursing but currently active working nurses

____ disillusioned with nursing and currently inactive, non-working nurses

____ active nurses still interested in nursing but wanting to expand the skills they bring to their practice

____ Other (please be specific) __________________________

____

____

____

(D) IN YOUR BEST ESTIMATION, NURSE-RECRUITS FOR NURSE PRACTITIONER PROGRAMS ARE PRIMARILY WHICH OF THE FOLLOWING TYPES; PLEASE CHECK JUST ONE RESPONSE.

____ disillusioned with nursing but currently active working nurses

____ disillusioned with nursing and currently inactive, non-working nurses

____ active nurses still interested in nursing but wanting to expand the skills they bring to their practice

____ Other (please be specific) ____________________

____

____

____

(7) IDENTIFYING VARIABLES ASSOCIATED WITH THE ACCEPTANCE OR REJECTION OF BOTH THE PA AND THE NP BY OTHER HEALTH PROFESSIONALS IS OF THE UTMOST CONCERN TO THOSE WHO ARE INVOLVED IN THEIR EDUCATION.

(A) WHAT FACTORS HAVE YOU FOUND TO BE THE MOST IMPORTANT IN PROMOTING THE ACCEPTABILITY OF THE PA AND/OR NP BY EXISTING MEDICAL AND OTHER HEALTH PROFESSIONALS? PLEASE RANK ORDER THE FOUR MOST IMPORTANT FACTORS ACCORDING TO THE FOLLOWING SCALE:

1 = most important
2 = second most important
3 = third most important
4 = fourth most important

____ the ability to do a demonstrably 'good' job, i.e., evidence maturity, intelligence, initiative, and concern for their patients.

____ a commitment to the concept of a team approach to patient care; included in this orientation should be a willingness to recognize the physician as the leader of the team and thus be willing to play a supportive role.

____ the PA and/or NP must understand and accept their roles in the provision of health care; the tasks assigned to them must not substitute for, or compete with, the tasks normally delegated to other health care professionals.

____ PAs and/or NPs working in a specialty area which is one of the most severely affected by the health manpower shortage (e.g., family practice) will be the most readily accepted by other health care professionals.

____ PAs and/or NPs willing to work in geographical areas which are suffering from a particularly severe health manpower shortage (e.g., some rural areas, urban ghettos) will be the most readily accepted by other health care professionals.

____ sufficient flexibility in defining the PA and/or NP role and general job description is important in order to allow maximum usage by their physician-employers and thus promote their acceptability by making them 'indispensable' to the physician.

____ PAs with a nursing background as well as NPs, who by definition are nurses, will be the most readily accepted since nurses are already an accepted and essential part of the health care system.

____ endorsement by the major health professions' organizations (e.g., AMA, ANA) will be the most important factor in promoting the acceptability of both of these new health workers by the other health professionals.

____ Other (please be specific) ________________________
____
____
____

(B) WHAT FACTORS HAVE YOU FOUND TO BE THE MOST DAMAGING TO EFFECTIVELY PROMOTING THE ACCEPTABILITY OF THE PA OR NP BY EXISTING MEDICAL AND OTHER HEALTH PROFESSIONALS? PLEASE RANK ORDER THE FOUR MOST DAMAGING FACTORS ACCORDING TO THE FOLLOWING SCALE:

1 = most important
2 = second most important
3 = third most important
4 = fourth most important

____ professional jealousy issues will hinder the acceptance of the PA and NP by existing professionals; i.e., the PA and NP will be viewed as 'intruders into nursing's territory.'

____ competition between employers (physicians) and employees (PA or NP) may develop; i.e., PAs and NPs may be viewed as 'more approachable,' by patients, than physicians; therefore, the physician may feel that a PA or NP would ultimately threaten his doctor-patient relationships rather than promote them.

____ physicians are too independent and will be unwilling to delegate enough challenging tasks to the PA or NP to make their roles meaningful ones; in addition, if the physician fails to utilize the PA or NP adequately, he may fail to see the importance of their potential contribution to better patient care.

____ economic arrangements may give rise to professional conflict; i.e., the RN may feel the NP or PA is comparatively 'overpaid' while the physician may resent having to pay more for the services of a PA or NP than he presently does for his regular office nurses.

____ failure to promote adequate understanding of the job the PA or NP is educated to fulfill will hinder their acceptance by the existing health establishment; this would include misunderstandings on the part of both the new health professionals and that of the existing health providers (e.g., nurse, physician).

____ lack of sufficient numbers of these new health professionals to make a dramatic enough impact on the health manpower situation in order to make the trauma associated with change tolerable; advocating change without demonstrating results is always ultimately met with antagonism.

____ fear of added insurance liability (e.g., higher premiums as well as greater risks associated with the use of a new health worker) may well cause physicians and hospitals to question the need for and/or lead to the underutilization of the PA and NP; both of these outcomes would be detrimental to the ultimate acceptance of the two new health professionals.

____ continuance of obsolete state medical practice acts which would unduly prevent adequate latitude for the growth of the PA and NP concepts would have obvious implications for damaging the acceptability of these workers.

____ Other (please be specific) ______________________

____

____

____

(8) IDENTIFYING VARIABLES ASSOCIATED WITH THE ACCEPTANCE OR REJECTION OF BOTH THE PA AND THE NP BY THE GENERAL PUBLIC IS ALSO OF THE UTMOST CONCERN TO THOSE WHO ARE INVOLVED IN THE EDUCATION OF THESE MEDICAL-ALLIED HEALTH PROFESSIONALS.

(A) WHAT FACTORS HAVE YOU FOUND TO BE THE MOST IMPORTANT IN PROMOTING THE ACCEPTABILITY OF THE PA OR THE NP BY THE GENERAL PUBLIC? PLEASE RANK ORDER THE FOUR MOST IMPORTANT FACTORS ACCORDING TO THE FOLLOWING SCALE:

1 = most important
2 = second most important
3 = third most important
4 = fourth most important

____ attention must be given to educating the general public as to the need for increased health manpower and the manner in which the PA and NP are to be used to help meet this need; only if the public is knowledgeable will they be willing to financially support, and accept the use of, the PA and the NP.

____ existing medical and other health professionals must actively promote the PA and NP concepts both to the general lay public and to their specific patients.

____ if the use of the PA or NP will lead to a reduction in the cost of medical care, the patient will be most likely to accept them as a vital part of the health care system.

____ the quality of care which the PA and the NP offer the public, as evidenced by maturity, commitment, and intelligence, will be the deciding factor in promoting the acceptance of their care by the public.

____ time is the crucial variable in promoting the acceptance of the PA and NP; the longer the NP and PA are active in the health field, the greater will be the public's acceptance.

____ if the PA and NP make available an increasing number of health services generally desired (e.g., home visits) but often not now available due to the health manpower shortage, the public will gratefully accept these new health professionals.

____ most important in promoting the acceptance of the PA and NP will be strong national support including not only sporadic rhetoric but active promotion of the idea through the mass media as well as financial support of educational programs and pilot demonstration projects.

____ Other (please be specific) ________________________
____
____
____

(B) WHAT FACTORS HAVE YOU FOUND TO BE THE MOST DAMAGING TO EFFECTIVELY PROMOTING THE ACCEPTABILITY OF THE PA OR THE NP BY THE GENERAL PUBLIC? PLEASE RANK ORDER THE THREE MOST IMPORTANT FACTORS ACCORDING TO THE FOLLOWING SCALE:

1 = most important
2 = second most important
3 = third most important

____ fear of obtaining 'inferior care' or 'second-class' medicine will unduly hamper the acceptance of the PA or NP by the public.

____ patients may fear that the PA or NP will interfere unduly with their primary relationship with the physician; patients want to communicate their problems directly to their physician and will resent this intermediary between them and the physician.

____ patients are unwilling to discuss their personal medical and emotional problems with anyone other than a physician.

____ patients may fear that their physician will use the PA or NP to increase the number of patients he cares for and thus increase his income rather than using the extra time for their benefit (e.g., devoting more time to the seriously ill).

____ patients tend to view their physician as a general family counselor; only after they have established a good relationship with their physician while they are 'in good health' are they willing to trust their physician to care for them when they are very ill; if their physician employs a NP or a PA to care for their 'routine ills,' they may feel that they would never get to see, much less know, their physician until they are already ill.

____ Other (please be specific) ______________________________
____
____
____

(9) LEGAL PROBLEMS ASSOCIATED WITH THE USE OF A PA OR NP HAVE BEEN CITED AS POTENTIAL OBSTACLES TO THE ACCEPTANCE AND FULL UTILIZATION OF THESE NEW HEALTH PROFESSIONALS. ALTHOUGH THERE ARE MANY SIMILARITIES IN THE TYPES OF LEGAL PROBLEMS WHICH WILL BE FACED BY BOTH THE PA AND THE NP, THERE ARE MANY UNIQUE ASPECTS OF THE ISSUES WHICH ARE APPLICABLE TO ONE OR THE OTHER OF THESE TWO CAREERS BUT NOT TO BOTH; FOR EXAMPLE, THE NP IS ALREADY A LICENSED PRACTITIONER WHO NOW WISHES TO EXPAND HER ROLE WHILE THE PA IS CONSIDERED TO BE A COMPLETELY NEW HEALTH CAREER WITHOUT PRIOR LICENSURE STATUS.

PLEASE NOTE CAREFULLY WHETHER THE QUESTIONS BELOW ARE DIRECTED TOWARD THE LEGAL PROBLEMS OF THE PHYSICIAN'S ASSISTANT OR THE NURSE PRACTITIONER AND THEN ANSWER WITH REFERENCE TO THE RELEVANT GROUP. FOR EXAMPLE, PA PROGRAMS WOULD ANSWER QUESTIONS REGARDING POTENTIAL LEGAL PROBLEMS OF NPs ON THE BASIS OF HOW THEY (PA PROGRAMS) FEEL THESE ISSUES WILL BE RESOLVED FOR NPs.

(A) WHAT DO YOU FEEL IS THE MOST LIKELY AND MOST POTENTIALLY DAMAGING LEGAL PROBLEM WHICH COULD IMPEDE THE FULL USE OF PHYSICIAN'S ASSISTANTS BY THE MEDICAL PROFESSION? PLEASE CHOOSE ONLY ONE RESPONSE.

____ criminal suits; the PA may be accused of practicing medicine without a license and his physician- or institution-employer may be accused of aiding and abetting such unlawful practice.

____ civil suits involving the doctrine of respondeat superior; i.e., the physician- or institution-employer may not be willing to assume responsibility for negligent acts committed by this new allied health professional; the use of a PA does not yet have the aura of legitimacy afforded by 'common custom and usage'; therefore, fear of taking on this added liability may make many physicians unwilling to hire PAs.

____ civil suits involving the doctrine of negligence per se; this would apply to both the PA and his physician- or institution-employer if injury resulted from an act committed in violation of an existing statute (e.g., medical practice act) without regard to the actual skill or competence with which the care was given; such violation could be found to exist solely on the basis of delegation of tasks to, or the performance of tasks by, unlicensed personnel.

____ Other (please be specific) ______________________________
____
____
____

(B) WHAT DO YOU FEEL IS THE MOST LIKELY AND MOST POTENTIALLY DAMAGING LEGAL PROBLEM WHICH COULD IMPEDE THE FULL USE OF NURSE PRACTITIONERS? PLEASE CHOOSE ONLY ONE RESPONSE.

____ criminal suits; the NP may be accused of practicing 'medicine' without a license while her physician- or institution-employer would be accused of aiding and abetting such unlawful practice.

____ civil suits involving the doctrine of respondeat superior; this doctrine holds regardless of licensure; the physician- or institution-employer, although willing to assume responsibility for negligent acts of his traditional nurse-employees, may be unwilling to assume like responsibility when she is functioning in an expanded role and possibly performing many tasks traditionally thought to be in the province of medicine. This may be particularly a problem if the nurse practice acts do not specifically allow the the NP's expanded functions under her regular license.

____ civil suits involving the doctrine of negligence per se; i.e., the NP, along with her physician- or institution-employer, may be accused of violation of both a state's nurse practice act (i.e., performing tasks which are beyond the scope of her nursing license and which are not officially recognized as being within the purview of nurses' competence as established by 'custom and usage') and the state's medical practice act (i.e., performing or delegating 'medical' tasks which are not officially exempted under the act), regardless of the skill or competence with which such care is given. Again, the charge of negligence per se does not depend upon the showing of actual negligence; one need only show that the person is functioning beyond the scope of their license and is thus considered 'unlicensed' to perform these particular tasks.

_____ although some cite the vagueness and ambiguity of nurse practice acts as supportive of the nurses' expanded role as a NP, this same vagueness and ambiguity may prove to be legally dangerous; delegation of health tasks is essentially governed by accepted 'custom and usage' which is very difficult to defend and document in a court of law; in addition, the NP has many new functions which are not traditionally considered to be part of the nurses' role and therefore could not adequately be defended under 'custom and usage.'

_____ Other (please be specific) ______________________________
____
____
____

(C) THE 1970 NATIONAL ACADEMY OF SCIENCES' REPORT ON THE PHYSICIAN'S ASSISTANT SUGGESTED THAT THE 'TYPE A' PHYSICIAN'S ASSISTANT COULD EXERCISE "A SMALL DEGREE OF INDEPENDENT MEDICAL JUDGMENT." HOW WOULD YOU INTERPRET THIS PHRASE? WHAT LEGAL IMPLICATIONS COULD THE USE OF SUCH 'INDEPENDENT MEDICAL JUDGMENT' HAVE?

(10) A 1972 MODEL LEGISLATION PROJECT, HELD IN NORTH CAROLINA, CONSIDERED SEVERAL ALTERNATIVES FOR RECOGNIZING THE LEGAL STATUS OF PHYSICIAN'S ASSISTANTS. NO FINAL AGREEMENT WAS REACHED IN SUPPORT OF A SPECIFIC ALTERNATIVE OR COMBINATION OF ALTERNATIVES; HOWEVER, THREE PROPOSALS WERE FELT TO HOLD EQUAL PROMISE OF PROVIDING AT LEAST A SATISFACTORY INTERIM MEASURE DURING WHICH THE ENTIRE LICENSURE ISSUE COULD BE STUDIED.

SECTIONS (A) AND (B) OF THIS QUESTION RELATE SPECIFICALLY TO RECOGNIZING THE LEGAL STATUS OF PHYSICIAN'S ASSISTANTS AND NOT NURSE PRACTITIONERS. NURSE PRACTITIONER PROGRAMS SHOULD ANSWER HOW THEY FEEL THE LEGAL ISSUES WILL, OR SHOULD BE, RESOLVED FOR THE PHYSICIAN'S ASSISTANT.

SECTION (C) OF THIS QUESTION RELATES SPECIFICALLY TO RECOGNIZING THE LEGAL STATUS OF NURSE PRACTITIONERS AND NOT PHYSICIAN'S ASSISTANTS. PHYSICIAN'S ASSISTANT PROGRAMS SHOULD ANSWER HOW THEY FEEL THE LEGAL ISSUES WILL, OR SHOULD BE, RESOLVED FOR THE NURSE PRACTITIONER.

(A) THE INITIAL SIX ALTERNATIVES FOR RECOGNIZING THE LEGAL STATUS OF THE PHYSICIAN'S ASSISTANT CONSIDERED AT THE 1972 MEETING ARE PRESENTED BELOW; OF THE SIX, WHICH DO YOU FEEL WOULD BE THE MOST EFFECTIVE AT THIS TIME? WHICH DO YOU FEEL WOULD PROVIDE THE BEST BASIS FOR A LONG-RANGE SOLUTION?

1 = most effective at this time
2 = best basis for a long-range solution

____ maintain the status quo; custom and usage, along with the assurance that the PA will remain in a dependent relationship to his physician- or institution-employer, will eventually afford the PA and the physician and institution sufficient legal protection.

____ license the PA in a manner similar to the licensure of other health professionals.

____ license the users of PAs; under this approach, the responsible licensing board would establish licensing criteria which physicians and/or institutions, desiring to hire an unlicensed PA, would have to meet before employing such personnel. This procedure would have to be followed each time a physician or institution wanted to hire a specific PA. A variation of this approach would allow the prospective employer to submit to the relevant licensing board(s) job descriptions for potential PA positions; upon approval of these job descriptions, the board(s) would set the qualifications necessary for an individual to assume these jobs. The user could then employ people who met these qualifications.

____ establish a multidisciplinary Committee on Health Manpower Innovations, under the auspices of the state medical board, which would review proposals for the training of new types of health manpower and provide legal sanction for the use of such personnel during the period of experimentation and before such use is validated through 'custom and usage' or more formal regulation.

____ authorize 'general delegations' by a physician to his 'trained assistant, a registered nurse, or a licensed practical nurse if such service be rendered under the direct supervision and control of the licensed physician'; this would prevent the PA and the physician from being accused of violation of licensure laws per se.

____ after providing an exemption clause under the state's medical practice act to allow the use of a PA, both the employer and the PA to be employed would have to be reviewed by the State Board of Medical Examiners; at a later date, a separate committee would be organized (under the State Board of Medical Examiners) to devise definitions for the scope of permissible practice for the PA as well as defining what constitutes 'proper' delegation by the physician; at a still later date, an independent multidisciplinary board or committee would be established to oversee the practice of all allied health professionals.

____ Other (please be specific) ____________________

____

____

____

(B) THE FOLLOWING THREE PROPOSALS WERE FELT BY THOSE ATTENDING THE 1972 CONFERENCE TO HOLD THE MOST PROMISE FOR THE RESOLUTION OF THE LEGAL QUESTIONS SURROUNDING THE USE OF THE PHYSICIAN'S ASSISTANT. PLEASE INDICATE WHICH ONE YOU WOULD FAVOR.

____ the October Proposal: (1) provide an exemption clause to the medical practice act so that delegation of medical functions, supervised and directed by a physician licensed by a Board of Medical Examiners, could be made by a physician to a physician's assistant provided the PA is approved by the Board of Medical Examiners in that state; (2) implicit in the Board's power of approval would be the power to deny or revoke such privilege when indicated; (3) the Board would develop guidelines to ensure that the appropriate degree of direction and supervision applicable to the particular situation and circumstances would govern the actions of both the PA and the physician and/or institution with whom he works; (4) the individual physician would have two functions: to evaluate his PA's capabilities and delegate accordingly and to provide 'adequate direction' and supervision. This proposal would not require a strict employer-employee relationship between physician and a physician's assistant; i. e., the PA's salary may be paid by a hospital although his activities must be under the direction and supervision of a licensed physician. In addition, since the PA will be delegated tasks traditionally performed only by a physician, the PA's performance of these tasks must be up to the standard and quality of the physician's performance of these same tasks.

____ the Havighurst Proposal: This proposal is very similar to the October Proposal in that it provides for an exemption clause to the medical practice act; however, it differs in two respects. It does not refer specifically to physician's assistants; rather, it allows delegation, by and under the supervision of a physician, of tasks to 'a person qualified by formal or informal training and experience to perform such tasks.' Secondly, the Board is not given prime responsibility in approving the prospective employee; primary reliance is placed on the employing physician or institution; the Board would oversee the actions of physicians and their assistants by investigating complaints concerning improper delegations and/or the performance of these tasks by inadequately prepared assistants.

____ the Hershey Proposal: This proposal is also similar to the above two proposals in that it is based on an exemption clause added to the state's medical practice act. Like the Havighurst proposal, it does not refer specifically to physician's assistants; rather, it allows a licensed physician to designate functions, specified in a Board approved job description, to a person who meets the Board approved qualifications for the job. As always, the licensed physician is responsible for directing and supervising the tasks performed by this person. It would be the responsibility of the physician to submit a detailed job description to the Board. With or without the physician's assistance, the Board would establish the necessary qualifications which the proposed employee must meet prior to employment. Although this proposal focuses on the primary role of the physician-employer and his licensing board, a similar procedure could be established for the supervision of assistant positions in institutions.

____ Other (please be specific) ______________________
____
____
____
____
____

(C) SOME THOUGHT HAS BEEN GIVEN TO RECOGNIZING THE LEGAL STATUS OF THE NURSE PRACTITIONER. OF THE FOLLOWING POSSIBLE COURSES OF ACTION, WHICH DO YOU FEEL WOULD BE THE MOST EFFECTIVE AT THIS TIME? WHICH DO YOU FEEL WOULD PROVIDE THE BEST BASIS FOR A LONG-RANGE SOLUTION?

1 = most effective at this time
2 = best basis for a long-range solution

____ maintain the status quo; i.e., allow the NP to function under her present registered nurse license. This assumes that the current nurse practice acts, without revision, are sufficiently vague and allow wide latitude in the nature of services rendered by the nurse so that a NP, functioning in an expanded capacity, would be legally protected by her present license.

____ a registered nurse can be delegated any medical procedure that does not, on a scientifically determined basis, require the personal knowledge, skill, and judgment of a physician. Therefore, to provide legal protection to the NP, one needs only to objectively evaluate medical tasks to determine which tasks require medical judgment and which do not; the latter could be safely delegated to the NP without fear of legal problems.

____ in order to adequately protect an RN who is prepared and functioning as a NP, there must be an explicit expansion of the tasks now allowed under state nurse practice acts; in particular, such acts should be amended to include more explicit provision for the nurse to perform tasks in physical diagnosis and patient care management.

____ Nurses completing nationally accredited nurse practitioner programs should be required to write a special licensure examination; upon successfully passing the exam, the nurse would, in effect, receive a second license. This special license would provide legal protection for the NP's expanded role in diagnosis, treatment, and some prescription.

____ Other (please be specific) ______________________________
____
____
____

(11) LICENSURE FOR THE PHYSICIAN'S ASSISTANT HAS BEEN A SOURCE OF SUBSTANTIAL DEBATE; A 1971 DHEW REPORT URGED A TWO-YEAR MORATORIUM ON LICENSURE OF ANY NEW HEALTH PERSONNEL DURING WHICH TIME THE ADVANTAGES AND DISADVANTAGES OF LICENSURE WOULD BE SUBJECTED TO INDEPTH STUDY.

IN ANSWERING THIS QUESTION, NURSE PRACTITIONER PROGRAMS SHOULD BASE THEIR RESPONSE ON WHAT THEY FEEL THE ADVANTAGES AND DISADVANTAGES OF LICENSING THE PHYSICIAN'S ASSISTANT WOULD BE.

(A) WHAT DOES YOUR PROGRAM FEEL WOULD BE THE MAJOR ADVANTAGES OF LICENSING THE PHYSICIAN'S ASSISTANT? PLEASE RANK ORDER TWO MAJOR ADVANTAGES ACCORDING TO THE FOLLOWING SCALE:

1 = major advantage
2 = second major advantage

____ licensing the PA would protect the PA and his physician-and/or institution-employer from charges of civil and criminal liability; liability would still naturally exist in cases of proven negligence and in cases where the PA was found to be functioning beyond the scope of his license.

____ licensure would enhance the status of the PA by recognizing it as a legitimate medical-allied health profession; this would promote the recruitment of career-oriented personnel as well as foster the acceptance of the PA by other health professionals and by the general public.

____ licensure of the PA would protect the public by insuring at least minimum qualifications and by officially delineating the new health professionals' areas of expertise; changes in scope of the PA's expertise could be accommodated by subsequent amendments to existing licensure legislation.

____ licensure of the PA would promote the geographic mobility of this new health worker; with his own license, the PA could more easily choose (or change) his employer (physician or institution) and geographic place of residence; the latter would assume the existence of provisions for licensure reciprocity among the states.

____ There are no advantages to licensing the PA.

____ Other (please be specific) ____________________

____

____

____

(B) WHAT DOES YOUR PROGRAM FEEL ARE THE MAJOR DISADVANTAGES OF LICENSING THE PHYSICIAN'S ASSISTANT? PLEASE RANK ORDER THREE MAJOR DISADVANTAGES ACCORDING TO THE FOLLOWING SCALE:

1 = major disadvantage
2 = second major disadvantage
3 = third major disadvantage

____ licensure is too restrictive for the newly evolving PA role; licensure would sharply limit the natural evolution of this new career and thus diminish the potential contribution of this approach designed to at least partially alleviate the health manpower shortage.

____ licensure of the PA would encourage fragmentation of health care delivery by reinforcing sharp (and often functionally irrelevant) boundaries between each of the medical-allied health professions.

____ licensure of the PA would sharply restrict occupational mobility (both vertical and lateral) by setting rigid formal educational requirements for entry into the field.

____ licensure would only perpetuate the 'guild system' of medicine; by licensing the PA, he will more readily become a part of the established health hierarchy; it is the established health hierarchy which needs to be changed; the PA should be a tool for making the needed changes in the system—not accommodate himself to the system!

____ licensure is inappropriate since the PA is a dependent profession and thus its independence as a separate medical-allied health profession ought to be controlled.

____ to develop an adequate license for the PA may well prove to be an impossible task; the functional sphere of a PA is determined by the setting in which he works (hospital, office, clinic), his employer (general practice physician, specialty physician, institution), and his formal educational and/or informal experience-related qualifications; conceivably there could be as many types of PAs as there are possible combinations of these functional sphere variables.

____ There are no disadvantages to licensing the PA.

____ Other (please be specific) ______________________________

____
____
____

(12) THE COST OF HEALTH CARE HAS RISEN RAPIDLY IN THE LAST DECADE. IF, AND IN WHAT MANNER, THESE COSTS ARE AFFECTED BY THE USE OF PAs AND NPs MAY DETERMINE THE ULTIMATE IMPACT THESE MEDICAL-ALLIED HEALTH PROFESSIONALS WILL MAKE ON OUR HEALTH CARE SYSTEM.

(A) WHAT EFFECT DOES YOUR PROGRAM FEEL THE USE OF THE PA AND THE NP WILL HAVE ON THE COST OF MEDICAL CARE TO THE PATIENT?

____ increase the cost ____ decrease the cost

____ no appreciable effect on cost

(B) GIVEN YOUR RESPONSE IN SECTION (A) OF THIS QUESTION, WHY DOES YOUR PROGRAM FEEL THAT THE USE OF THE PA AND NP WILL AFFECT THE COST OF MEDICAL CARE TO THE PATIENT IN THE MANNER INDICATED?

(C) APPROXIMATE ANNUAL SALARY OF YOUR GRADUATES? $____

(D) ESTIMATED COST OF TRAINING EACH OF YOUR GRADUATES? $____

(13) BRIEFLY, PLEASE COMMENT ON YOUR PROGRAM'S SUCCESS IN PROVIDING THE NATION WITH NEW HIGHLY SKILLED MEDICAL-ALLIED HEALTH PROFESSIONALS.

(A) IN WHAT TYPES OF POSITIONS HAVE YOUR GRADUATES BEEN PLACED?

(B) DO YOU HAVE ANY KNOWLEDGE OF THE ACCEPTABILITY OF YOUR GRADUATES IN THEIR NEW POSITIONS BY THE PHYSICIANS, OTHER HEALTH PROFESSIONALS, AND PATIENTS WITH WHOM THEY WORK?

(C) WHAT APPEAR TO BE YOUR GRADUATES' MOST POSITIVE AND MOST NEGATIVE ATTRIBUTES?

Positive:

Negative:

(14) WHAT SINGLE PROBLEM DOES YOUR PROGRAM FEEL IS THE MOST IMPORTANT ONE TO RESOLVE IN ORDER TO EFFECTIVELY PROMOTE THE WIDESPREAD USE OF PHYSICIAN'S ASSISTANTS AND/OR NURSE PRACTITIONERS?

(15) AS AN EDUCATIONAL PROGRAM EVOLVES, GOALS, OBJECTIVES, CURRICULUM, ETC... ARE CONSTANTLY SUBJECTED TO EVALUATION AND REFORMULATION. AS YOUR PROGRAM HAS GROWN, WHAT CHANGES HAVE OCCURRED IN YOUR PROGRAM'S CONCEPTION OF THE 'IDEAL' PA OR NP? WHAT WAS THE IMPETUS FOR THESE CHANGES? HOW HAS THIS CHANGED PERCEPTION OF THE

PA OR NP ROLE LED TO THE RESTRUCTURING OF YOUR GOALS AND PROGRAM CURRICULUM? (Short Concise Phrases Would Be Fine)

(16) IN THIS FINAL QUESTION, WE WOULD LIKE TO OBTAIN SOME GENERAL BACKGROUND INFORMATION ON YOUR PROGRAM.

(A) THE FUNCTIONAL STATUS OF YOUR PROGRAM:

(1) Is your program in the planning or operational stage of development?

____ planning stage ____ operational stage

(2) Length of planning stage (in months and/or years)

____

(3) Length of operational stage (in months and/or years)

____

(B) GENERAL PROGRAM INFORMATION:

(1) Educational Base for your program:

____ medical school ____ federal institution

____ junior or community college ____ medical center

____ 4-year college or university ____ Other (please be specific) ________ ________________

(2) Pre-requisite for entrance: ______________________________

(3) Length of educational program (both didactic and clinical):

____ didactic ____ clinical

(4) Patient group your program is primarily designed to serve:

_____ urban ghetto _____ rural poor

_____ general population, all income groups

_____ medically-underserved rural area, all income groups

_____ 'special' population with particular health needs such as children, elderly, pregnant women, etc...; all income groups are represented; please specify special group ______________________________

_____ Other (please be specific) ______________________
____

(5) Settings in which your graduate is capable of working:

_____ private physician's office, responsible to a single physician in the practice

_____ private physicians' office, responsible to entire group of physicians in the practice

_____ general community; i.e., schools, home visits

_____ outpatient clinics, with physician present at all times

_____ outpatient clinics, physician need not be physically present

_____ hospital

_____ extended care facility

_____ mental health clinic

_____ public health department

_____ Other (please be specific) ______________________
____
____

(C) THE IMPETUS FOR THE PROGRAM:

(1) Did the initial impetus for the program originate in an

institution of higher learning? Which colleges and/or departments were primarily involved?

(2) What type of active community support for the program was shown initially and as the program evolved? For example, was the local community hospital involved or was involvement restricted to university-affiliated hospitals?

(3) Which professional associations were most actively involved in the initial stages of the program? In what ways did they manifest their support (or lack of support) for the program?

(4) Which level of government was most helpful in the initiation of your program (e.g., funding, technical assistance)?

____ federal ____ state ____ regional ____ local

____ no governmental assistance

(5) Is there any state and/or regional comprehensive health planning agency in your area? What assistance (if any) have you received from this agency in the planning and implementing of your program?

(6) Approximate number of current students: ______________

(7) Approximate number of graduates: ______________

(8) Approximate number of graduates currently employed as PAs or NPs: ______________

(9) Approximate ratio of males to females in total student and graduate population of your program: ______________

(10) Approximate ratio of Black, Indian, Chicano to White in total student and graduate population of your program:

____

(11) Average age of your program's recruits: ____________

(12) Award upon graduation:

____ certificate ____ Associate degree

____ Baccalaureate ____ Master's

(13) Are your graduates eligible for some type of license? Please specify type of license.

____ Yes: Type ____ ____ No

(D) GENERAL INFORMATION ON RESPONDENT:

(1) Educational and professional degrees: ____________

(2) Position in the program: ____________

(3) Length of time with the program: ____________

APPENDIX C

PHYSICIAN QUESTIONNAIRE: LOCAL STUDY, 1970

Name:

Address:

Age:

Medical School (Name and Location): Area of Specialization:

Hometown:

No. of years of practice in this city:

In recent years, many have decried the shortage of physicians. One potential solution to the physician shortage has been the development of a new type of health professional called the physician's assistant. A 1970 report of the Board on Medicine of the National Academy of Sciences divided the broader concept of the physician's assistant into three definitive categories of personnel; in essence, these three categories reflect different grades of physician's assistants.

(a) The <u>physician's associate</u> - This individual is the most highly trained type of physician's assistant. He would be capable of assisting the physician by performing diagnostic and therapeutic procedures (under the physician's general supervision) and coordinating the roles of other, more technical, assistants. While he would function under the general supervision and responsibility of the physician, he might (under special circumstances) perform without the <u>immediate</u> surveillance of the physician. He may be expected to exercise a small degree of independent medical judgment.

(b) The <u>specialist assistant</u> - This individual is highly skilled in one type of clinical specialty <u>or</u> procedure within a specialty. Although he has a limited area of knowledge and skill, he has a depth of training and skill within this area which is exceeded only by the specialist-physician working within the same field.

He is less capable of independent action than the physician's associate.

(c) The nonspecialized assistant - This individual would be capable of performing a variety of tasks over the whole range of medical care under the supervision of a physician with whom this assistant would work in close proximity. He does not have the level of knowledge necessary to integrate and interpret the findings he has obtained in his testing of the patient. Generally his training is less formal than that of either the physician's associate or specialist assistant; much of his training is obtained by on-the-job experience with the physician for whom he will work.

Although it is not specifically stated in the above definition, assume that all of the above could be educated to function as an assistant to the obstetrician; please answer the questions with this in mind. Unless specified, please answer each question with the one best response.

(1) As a practicing obstetrician in this area, do you feel that there is a need for any of the above categories of physician's assistants here?

Yes ____ No ____

(2) (A) Rank the three types of physician's assistants mentioned above according to how useful you feel they would be to you in your practice; i.e., 1 = most useful.

(a) ____ (b) ____ (c) ____

(B) With regard to the one type which you rated as 'most useful', indicate why you feel this type of physician's assistant would be the most useful to you in your practice. (You may choose more than one answer.)

Most self-reliant ____ Most highly educated ____

Sufficient relevant education ____

Would work best and be most content in an assistant position ____

Other ____________________
(Please be specific)

(3) (A) If the type of physician's assistant (which you specified as 'most useful' in question 2) were available in this community, would you use one in your practice?

Yes ____ No ____

(B) If you said you would not use one, why do you feel this way? (Only one response please.)

Personally, I need no help of the assistant variety in my practice ________

Would take too much of my time supervising such an assistant ________

Other ____________
(Please be specific)

Not sufficient preparation to exercise any degree of independent medical judgment ________

Would be afraid of a malpractice suit since I would be responsible for his actions ________

(4) Are you opposed to the use of the physician's assistant in general? (One response.)

No, I would use a physician's assistant. ____

No; I do not want to use one myself but if another obstetrician wishes to do so, I am not opposed to his use of one. ____

Yes; I do not think the use of a physician's assistant is justified; its value has not been proven yet. ____

(5) Would you be willing to be the first obstetrician in this community to employ the services of an obstetrical physician's assistant?

Yes ____ No ____ Undecided ____

(6) Of the obstetricians in the city, which one would you most likely consult with regarding the advisability of using a physician's assistant in obstetrical practice?

____

(7) Do you feel that the shortage of obstetricians in this city is sufficiently acute to be termed a crisis situation?

Yes ____ No ____

(8) The development of a new type of health personnel always requires that the legal implications surrounding the practice of the new worker be resolved.

(A) What method do you think will be employed in order to resolve the legal implications of the use of 'medical judgment' by the physician's assistant? (One response.)

Legislative certification under the license of the physician for whom he works ________

Judicial test case to determine the degree of independent medical judgment permissible by the physician's assistant ______

Independent licensure of the physician's assistant, with control by malpractice ________

Other ________________
(Please be specific)

(B) What factors do you think will be most important in resolving the legal implications surrounding the use of the physician's assistant? (One response.)

Professional organization (e.g., AMA) and its political power will be important in resolving this issue ____________

Judicial test case re the independence of the physician's assistant as a separate profession in its own right and thus accountable for its own actions ____________

Judicial test case re the extent of independent medical judgment permissible by the physician's assistant ____________

Other ____________
(Please be specific)

(C) The last session of the State Legislature adopted an amendment to the Medical Practice Act for the State which concerned the use of physician's assistants. Are you aware of this amendment? What does the amendment entail?

Yes ____ No ____

(9) (A) How do you view the question of licensure for the physician's assistant?

Favor it ____

Do not favor it at this time; perhaps acceptable in the future ____

Never would favor it ____

(ANSWER EITHER B OR C OF QUESTION NUMBER 9 BASED ON YOUR ANSWER IN 9A)

(B) Why are you against licensure of the physician's assistant? (One response.)

Competitive with physician ____

Physician's assistants may become too independent if they had their own license ____

Physician's assistants are not a separate profession; therefore they should not have a separate license ____

Other ____________
(Please be specific)

(C) Why do you favor licensure of the physician's assistant? (One response.)

Licensure would imply minimum standards; thus licensure would be a way of controlling the education and practice of the physician's assistant ____

Other ____________
(Please be specific)

(D) Regardless of how you feel about licensure of the physician's assistant, do you feel that licensure of the physician's assistant will become an eventual reality?

Yes ____ No ____

(10) (A) If physician's assistants were to become licensed, do you feel that they would eventually be able to be hired by hospitals, such as nurses are today, under the auspices of a salaried hospital physician, or under the auspices of the hospital's medical board?

Yes ____ No ____

(B) If you answered No, why not? (One response.)

Physician's assistant will work best in a 1:1 relationship with a physician ____

Other ____________
(Please be specific)

If this happened, the physician's assistant could not be adequately controlled in his 'assistant' role; he would be practicing medicine ____

(11) Of potential recruitment sources for the physician's assistant programs, which of the following would be acceptable to you? (You may make more than one choice. Assume that all of the people, regardless of initial occupation or training, would be exposed to additional preparation in order to function as a physician's assistant.)

College graduate, with health-related major ____
College graduate, with non-health-related major ____
Nurse (RN), either male or female ____
Nurse (PN), either male or female ____
Hospital Technician (e.g., inhalation therapist) ____
High School graduate ____

(12) (A) Which one of the above recruitment sources would you favor?

____

(B) Why would you favor this recruitment source over the others? (You may make more than one response; however, place two checks by the one reason you feel is most important in your choice.)

more highly educated ________
more health-related educational background ____
more health-related practical experience ____
more likely to be willing to train for an 'assistant' type of occupation ________
already a health professional, accepted by the public and by the physicians ________

(13) The recent official ANA and NLN position with regard to the recruitment of physician's assistants from the ranks of nurses was very unfavorable; in essence, their position is that nurses are needed for nursing; nursing schools are not for the training of physician's assistants.

(A) What is your personal reaction to the ANA and NLN positions?

(B) If you chose the nurse in answer to question number 12, how would you resolve this question - in the light of the ANA's and the NLN's position?

(C) The AMA has recently taken an official position on the nurses' potential role as a physician's assistant. What is that position?

Don't know ____

(14) Would you prefer the physician's assistant (obstetrical physician's assistant) to be a male or would you prefer this career to be largely a female occupation?

Male ____ Female ____ Either ____

(15) Which professional organizations do you feel are relevant to you in helping you clarify your general opinions re the practice of medicine?

(B) Are you a member of the organization(s) which you named in 15A?

Yes ____ No ____

(16) (A) What leadership positions do you hold in this community? (Please include both medical and other community leadership roles (e.g., church).)

(B) What leadership positions do you hold outside this community? For example, chairmanship of the State Committee on .....

(17) How do you feel about the following:

	STRONGLY AGREE	AGREE	DISAGREE	STRONGLY DISAGREE
It is all right for the federal government to be involved in the education of physicians, but the federal government should not become more involved than it is in the delivery and/or subsidization of health care.	____	____	____	____
The physician of the future will probably be a salaried employee of a larger institution such as a hospital, a university, or the government.	____	____	____	____
There will always be a place for the 'solo' practitioner in medicine.	____	____	____	____
Specialty groups are an acceptable way to practice medicine, provided the individual physicians are responsible for its organization and functioning and not a third party such as the government.	____	____	____	____

(18) (A) Politically, how do you classify yourself? (One response.)

Conservative ____ Middle-of-the-road ____ Liberal ____

(B) In medical matters, how do you classify yourself?

Conservative ____ Middle-of-the-road ____ Liberal ____

(C) How would you classify your political activism? (One response.)

Passive voter ____ Moderately politically active (i.e., give money, aware of issues ____ Very politically active (i.e., actively work for issues and candidates ____

(19) In a few key phrases, what do you regard as the 'ideal' characteristics of a good physician? (You may check more than one; please place two checks beside the characteristic you feel is most important for a good physician.)

intellectually competent in his specialty ____

empathetic to his patients; concerned for their welfare ____

honest in his dealings with his patients ____

Other ________ (Please be specific)

loyal to his colleagues ____

'keeps up' with current medical knowledge in his field ____

is an 'all-round' well-educated person ____

active in his professional organization ____

(20) In a few key phrases, what do you regard as the 'ideal' characteristics of a good nurse? (You may check more than one response; please place two checks beside the characteristic you feel is most important for a good nurse.)

Efficient ____

satisfaction with her nurse's role ____

loyal to her colleagues and to the medical profession ____

genuine concern for patients' welfare ____

competent ____

Other ________ (Please be specific)

pleasant personality ____

able to question Dr.'s orders intelligently ____

(21) In a few key phrases, what do you regard as the 'ideal' characteristics of a good patient? (You may check more than one response; please place two checks beside the characteristic you feel is most important for a good patient.)

asks relevant questions ____

reports health problem promptly ____

pleasant personality ____

Other ________ (Please be specific)

carries out physician's orders faithfully ____

(22) What are your general feelings toward the usefulness of your present nurse assistant(s)? (You may check more than one response; however, please put two checks beside the response that best describes your general feelings toward your nurse assistant.)

indispensable ____

necessary to guard against malpractice ____

fairly helpful ____

adequately trained ____

would be more useful if she had more specialized training ____

Other ____________
(Please be specific)

(23) Generally, how do you think the new occupation of a physician's assistant in obstetrics would affect the role of the obstetrical nurse?

It would provide a new opportunity for the nurse to expand her role in obstetrics by obtaining just a little more training ____

I think the new job will be competitive with the nurses' role in obstetrics ____

I think the new job will interfere with the present doctor-nurse working relations in obstetrics; in effect, the nurse will have another boss ____

I think the new job will take away from the nurse many of the 'medical' functions which have, by default, fallen to the nurse ____

Other ____________
(Please be specific)

(24) If the new job of obstetrical physician's assistant will take away many of the functions now done by the obstetrical nurse, how would you feel about this change?

Would favor it for the nurse is needed more in other areas of health care than in obstetrics ____

Would favor it because many of the tasks which have fallen to the nurse are tasks which the nurse is not really adequate to handle____

Would not favor it; the nurse is fully capable of the tasks which she has assumed ____

Other ____________
(Please be specific)

(25) Which faction will be most influential in promoting the acceptability of the physician's assistant?

Individual physicians by their expressed demand ____ AMA ____ The public ____

(26) (A) What effect do you think the use of obstetrical physician's assistants will have on the cost of obstetrical care to the patient?

reduce it ____ no effect ____ may increase the cost of care ____

ANSWER EITHER B OR C OR D OF QUESTION NUMBER 26:

(B) Why do you think it will reduce the cost of obstetrical care to the patient?

(C) Why do you think it will increase the cost of obstetrical care to the patient?

(D) Why do you think it will have no effect on the cost of obstetrical care to the patient?

(27) What is your general attitude toward the use of a physician's assistant? What can you see as the prime advantages, and disadvantages, of the use of an obstetrical physician's assistant? (Please answer from the standpoint of a physician.)

If the functions performed by an obstetrician were broken down into the following tasks, which tasks would you delegate to a physician's assistant who worked with you?

TASK	STRONGLY FAVOR DELEGATION	FAVOR DELEGATION	DO NOT FAVOR DELEGATION	STRONGLY DO NOT FAVOR DELEGATION	TYPE (OR TYPES) OF P.A.* TO WHOM YOU WOULD DELEGATE THE TASK	DEGREE OF SUPERVISION YOU WOULD REQUIRE OF THE P. A. DELEGATED THE TASK**
Initial History & Physical						
Initial Pelvic Exam.						
Papanicolaou Smear						
Pelvimetry, Physical						
Routine Prenatal Care						
Lab Tests:						
Pregnancy Tests						
CBC						
Urinalysis						
Blood typing						
VDRL						
Coombs test						
Make Emergency Room Visits						
Take 'on call'						
Primary Rx for a woman with preeclampsia						
Follow-up treatment for a woman with preeclampsia						
Primary treatment for a woman with eclampsia						
Follow-up treatment for a woman with eclampsia						
Administer anesthesia (under physician's supervision)						
General						
Spinal						
Saddle block						
Pudendal						
Paracervical						

TASK	STRONGLY FAVOR DELEGATION	FAVOR DELEGATION	DO NOT FAVOR DELEGATION	STRONGLY DO NOT FAVOR DELEGATION	TYPE (OR TYPES) OF P.A. TO WHOM YOU WOULD DELEGATE THE TASK	DEGREE OF SUPERVISION YOU WOULD REQUIRE OF THE P. A. DELEGATED THE TASK
Assist with a C-Section						
Deliver normal primipara						
Deliver normal multipara						
Deliver a multiple birth						
Deliver a breech birth						
Manage routine post-partum care						
Administer intravenous therapy						
Do venous cut-downs						
Administer blood						
Do exchange transfusions in newborn						
Do intra-uterine fetal transfusions						
Do amniotic fluid evaluation						
Routine use of outlet forceps						
Conduct 6-week post-partum check-up						
Hospital visits post-partum						
Routine follow-up home visits post-partum						

*Types: A = Physician's associate
B = Specialist assistant
C = Nonspecialized assistant.

**High, moderate, or minimal supervision.

APPENDIX D

NURSE QUESTIONNAIRE: LOCAL STUDY, 1970

Name:

Address:

Age:

'Hometown':

Nursing School attended (name and location):

Type of nursing program:

Number of years in active nursing practice (any type of active nursing practice):

Any special preparation you have had in obstetrical nursing (i.e., midwifery training):

Number of years working in obstetrical nursing:

Physician(s) for whom you work:

In recent years, many have decried the shortage of physicians. One potential solution to the physician shortage has been the development of a new form of health professional called the physician's assistant. A recent report of the Board on Medicine of the National Academy of Sciences divided the broader concept of the physician's assistant into three more refined categories of personnel; in effect, these three categories reflect different grades of physician's assistants.

(a) The physician's associate - This individual is the most highly trained type of physician's assistant. He would be capable of assisting the physician by performing diagnostic and therapeutic procedures (under the physician's general supervision) and coordinating the roles of more technical assistants. While he would function under the general supervision and responsibility of the physician, he might (under special circumstances) perform without the immediate surveillance of the physician. He may be expected to exercise a small degree of independent medical judgment.

(b) The specialist assistant - This individual is highly skilled in one type of clinical specialty or procedure within a specialty. Although he has a limited area of knowledge and skill, he has a depth of training and skill within this area which is exceeded only by the specialist-physician working within the same field. He is less capable of independent action than the physician's associate.

(c) The nonspecialized assistant - This individual would be capable of performing a variety of tasks over the whole range of medical care, under the supervision of a physician with whom this assistant would work in close proximity. He does not have the level of knowledge necessary to integrate and interpret the findings he has obtained in his testing of the patient. Generally his training is less formal than that of either the physician's associate or specialist assistant; much of his training is obtained by on-the-job experience with the physician for whom he will work.

Although it is not specifically stated in the above definitions, assume that all of the above could be educated to function as an assistant to the obstetrician; please answer the questions with this in mind. Unless specified, please answer each question with the one best response.

---

(1) As a working obstetrical nurse, do you feel that there is a need for any of the above types of physician's assistants in this community?

Yes ____ No ____

(2) (A) Rank the three types of physician's assistants described above according to how useful you feel they would be in an obstetrician's office; i.e., 1 = most useful.

(a) ____ (b) ____ (c) ____

(B) With regard to the one type which you rated most useful to an obstetrician's practice, why do you feel this type would be most useful? (You may choose more than one response.)

most self-reliant ____

highest educated ____

sufficient relevant education ____

Other ____________
(Please be specific)

would work best and be most content in an assistant position ____

would best complement, and not compete with, the nurses' role in obstetrics ____

(3) Would you be willing to be the first obstetrical nurse in this community to engage in additional training in order to qualify as an obstetrical physician's assistant - and then to work here as such?

Yes ____ No ____ Undecided ____

(4) (A) Of the obstetrical nurses in this community (i.e., those who work either in obstetrician's offices or in the obstetrical services in the hospital), which one would (give name) you probably consult with regarding what the 'best' attitude toward the physician's assistant should be?

____________ (or) I would not consult a nurse; I would consult ____________, who is a ________________.

(B) Why would you consult this person?

personal friend ________

usually has more information than I in professional matters ____

Other ____________
(Please be specific)

(5) The development of a new type of health personnel always requires that the legal implications surrounding the practice of the new worker be resolved.

(A) What method do you think will be employed in order to resolve the legal implications of the use of 'medical judgment' by the physician's assistant? (One response please.)

Legislative certification under the license of the physician for whom he works ____

Independent licensure of the physician's assistant, with control by malpractice ____

Judicial test case to determine the degree of independent medical judgment permissible by the physician's assistant ____

Other ____________
(Please be specific)

(B) What factors do you think will be most important in resolving the legal implications surrounding the use of the physician's assistants? (One response.)

Professional organization (e.g., AMA) and its political power will be important in resolving this issue ____

Judicial test case re the extent of independent medical judgment permissible by the physician's assistant ____

Judicial test case re the independence of the physician's assistant as a separate profession in its own right and thus accountable for its own actions ____

Other ____________
(Please be specific)

(6) (A) How do you view the question of licensure for the physician's assistant?

Favor it ____	Do not favor it at this time; perhaps acceptable in the future ____	Never would favor it ____

(ANSWER EITHER B OR C OF QUESTION NUMBER 6 BASED ON YOUR ANSWER TO 6A)

(B) Why are you against licensure of the physician's assistant? (One response.)

potentially competitive with physician ____

potentially competitive with nurse ____

physician's assistants may become too independent if they had their own license ____

physician's assistants are not a separate established profession; therefore, they should not have a separate license ____

Other ___________
(Please be specific)

(C) Why do you favor licensure of the physician's assistant? (One response.)

licensure would imply minimum standards; thus licensure would be a way of controlling the education and practice of the physician's assistant ________

Other ___________
(Please be specific)

(D) Regardless of how you feel about the desirability of the physician's assistant being licensed, do you feel that licensure of the physician's assistant will become an eventual reality?

Yes ____ No ____

(7) If physician's assistants were to become licensed, do you feel that they would eventually be able to be hired by hospitals, such as nurses are today, under the auspices of a salaried hospital physician or under the auspices of the hospital's medical board?

Yes ____ No ____

(8) Of potential recruitment sources for the physician's assistant programs, which of the following would you think of as a good potential source for physician's assistants? (You may make more than one choice. Assume that all of the people, regardless of initial occupation or training, would be exposed to additional preparation in order to function as a physician's assistant.)

College graduate, with health-related major ____
College graduate, with non-health-related major ____
Nurse (RN), either male or female ____
Nurse (PN), either male or female ____
High School graduate ____
Hospital Technician (e.g., inhalation therapist) ____
Military Medic ____
Any, if all were trained in a qualified physician's assistant program ____

(9) (A) Which one of the above recruitment sources would you favor?

____

(B) Why would you favor this recruitment source over the others? (You may make more than one response; however, place two checks by the one reason you feel is most important in your choice.)

more highly educated ____

more health-related educational background ____

more likely to train for an 'assistant' type of occupation ____

already a health professional, accepted by the public and by the physicians ____

Other ____________
(Please be specific)

(10) The recent AMA's official position on 'Nursing and Medicine in the 70s' supported the role of the nurse as physician's assistant; she would have to take 'modest additional training' in order to qualify for the position of physician's assistant.

What is your personal reaction to the AMA's position?

(11) The ANA and the NLN recently issued a statement regarding their position on the proper role of the nurse and how it should relate to the physician's assistant. In essence, the position states that nurses are needed for nursing; nursing schools are not for the training of physician's assistants.

(A) What is your personal reaction to the ANA and NLN position?

(B) If you chose the nurse in answer to question number 9A, how would you resolve this issue conflict - in the light of the ANA and NLN position?

(12) Would you prefer the physician's assistant (obstetrical physician's assistant) to be a male or would you prefer this career to be largely a female occupation?

Male ____ Female ____ Either ____

(13) (A) Which professional organizations do you feel are relevant to you in helping you clarify your general opinions re the practice of medicine and/or nursing?

(B) Are you a member of the organization(s) which you named in 13A? What organizations are you a member of?

Yes ____ No ____

Names of organizations you are a member of ________

(14) (A) What leadership positions do you hold in this community? (Please include nursing-related as well as other community leadership roles such as in a church organization.)

(B) What leadership positions do you hold outside of the community? For example, chairmanship of a committee of the State chapter of ANA.

(15) How do you feel about the following:

	STRONGLY AGREE	AGREE	DISAGREE	STRONGLY DISAGREE
It is all right for the federal government to be involved in the education of physicians, but the federal government should not become more involved than it is in the delivery and/or subsidization of health care.	____	____	____	____
The physician of the future will probably be a salaried employee of a larger institution such as a hospital, a university, or the government.	____	____	____	____
There will always be a place for the 'solo' practitioner in medicine.	____	____	____	____

	STRONGLY AGREE	AGREE	DISAGREE	STRONGLY DISAGREE
Specialty groups are an acceptable way to practice medicine, provided the individual doctors are left responsible for its organization and functioning and not a third party such as the government.	____	____	____	____

(16) (A) Politically, how do you classify yourself? (One response)

Conservative ____ Middle-of-the-road ____ Liberal ____

(B) In nursing matters, how do you classify yourself?

Conservative ____ Middle-of-the-road ____ Liberal ____

(C) How would you classify your political activism?

Passive voter ____

Moderately politically active; i.e., give money, aware of issues ____

Very politically active; i.e., actively work for issues and candidates ____

(17) In a few key phrases, what do you regard as the 'ideal' characteristics of a good physician? (You may check more than one; however, please place two checks beside the characteristic you feel is most important for a good physician.)

intellectually competent in his specialty ____

empathetic to his patients; concerned about their welfare ____

honest in his dealings with his patients ____

loyal to his colleagues ____

'keeps up' with current medical knowledge in his field ____

is an 'all-round' well-educated person ____

active in his professional organization ____

Other ____________
(Please be specific)

(18) In a few key phrases, what do you regard as the 'ideal' characteristics of a good nurse? (You may check more than one response; however, please place two checks beside the characteristic you feel is most important for a good nurse.)

efficient ____

loyal to her colleagues and to the medical profession ____

competent ____

pleasant personality ____

satisfaction with her nurse's role ____

genuine concern for the patient's welfare ____

Other ____________
(Please be specific)

able to question physician's orders intelligently ____

(19) In a few key phrases, what do you regard as the 'ideal' characteristics of a good patient? (You may check more than one response; however, please place two checks beside the characteristic you feel is most important for a good patient to possess.)

asks relevant questions ____

pleasant personality ____

reports health problem promptly ____

carries out physician's orders faithfully ____

Other ____________
(Please be specific)

(20) What are your present feelings toward your role as an obstetrical nurse? (You may check more than one.)

I feel I am not really doing 'nursing' ____

I am satisfied with my position ____

The physician gives me a lot of responsibility ____

The physician does not give me enough responsibility ____

Other ____________
(Please be specific)

(21) Generally, how do you think the new occupation of physician's assistant in obstetrics would affect you as an obstetrical nurse? (Only one response.)

It would be a new opportunity for me to expand my role in obstetrics by obtaining just a little more training ____

I think the new job will be competitive with nursing ____

I think the new job would interfere with the present nurse-doctor working relationship; in effect, the nurse will have another boss ____

I think the new job will take away from the nurse many of the 'medical' functions which have, by default, fallen to the nurse ____

Other ____________

(22) If the new job of obstetrical physician's assistant will take away many of the functions now done by the obstetrical nurse, how would you feel about this change?

Would favor it for the nurse is needed more in other areas of health care than in obstetrics ____

Would favor it because many of the tasks which have fallen to the nurse are tasks which the nurse is not really trained to handle ____

Would not favor it; the nurse is fully capable of the tasks which she has assumed ____

Other ____________
(Please be specific)

(23) Which faction do you think will be most influential in promoting the acceptability of the physician's assistant?

Individual physicians by their expressed demand ____ AMA ____ The public ____

(24) (A) What effect do you think the use of obstetrical physician's assistants will have on the cost of obstetrical care to the patient?

reduce it ____ no effect ____ may increase the cost of care ____

ANSWER EITHER B OR C OR D OF QUESTION NUMBER 24:

(B) Why do you think it will reduce the cost of obstetrical care to the patient?

(C) Why do you think it will increase the cost of obstetrical care to the patient?

(D) Why do you think it will have no effect on the cost of obstetrical care to the patient?

(25) What is your general attitude toward the use of a physician's assistant? What can you see as the prime advantages, and disadvantages, of the use of an obstetrical physician's assistant? (Answer from the standpoint of an obstetrical nurse.)

APPENDIX E

PATIENT QUESTIONNAIRE: LOCAL STUDY, 1970

Name:
Address:
Age:
Occupation: employed ____
unemployed ____
Phone number:
Husband's occupation:
'Hometown':
Highest level of education actually completed in school (circle highest level): 1 2 3 4 5 6 7 8 9 10 11 12 College 1 2 3 4 5 6 7 8 9+
Obstetrician's name:
No. of previous pregnancies (not including present one):
Present month of this pregnancy:

In answering the following questions, attempt to sort out your own personal feelings toward your doctor. Many pregnant women tend to develop a very 'special' relationship with their obstetrician. Quite naturally, when women are pregnant and seeing their obstetrician regularly, they develop very definite opinions about their own doctor. If possible, attempt to answer these questions without reference to your own personal feelings about your own doctor; rather answer the questions in relation to how you think you would feel toward the new type of health worker we will be talking about, if you had begun to use him at the beginning of your pregnancy before you had developed any personal opinions about, or loyalty to, your own doctor.

Today many people are worried about the shortage of health workers that appears to exist in the United States. In particular, there has been much concern about the limited number of doctors available. In recent years, one possible solution to the limited number of doctors has been suggested. This solution is the development of a new type of health worker to 'help' the doctor give more care to more patients. This type of worker would be known as the physician's assistant. The type and extent of the physician's assistant's training and education would vary depending on what type of doctor the assistant worked with. (Assume in answering any of the questions in this questionnaire that the physician's assistant about which we will be talking has been adequately trained for his job.) A physician's assistant could be defined as an advanced health worker with special training, intermediate between that of a technician (such as an x-ray technician) and the doctor. He would generally have a more intensive medical knowledge than the nurse. The physician's assistant could handle many technical procedures and could take some degree of independent medical responsibility. For example, the physician's assistant may be responsible for giving you your initial physical examination to determine if you are pregnant; if, as a result of the examination, the assistant finds that there appears to be some problem, the doctor himself would then examine you to determine what should be done about the problem.

(1) If there were physician's assistants available in this community who were specially trained to take care of many of the needs of pregnant women, would you be willing to have them help the doctor take care of you during your pregnancy? (One response please.)

Yes ____ No ____ Undecided ____

(2) (A) Which sex would you prefer the physician's assistant to be? (One response.)

Female ____ Male ____ Either sex is equally acceptable ____ Neither sex since I would not use a physician's assistant ____

(B) Would you accept either sex equally well in the role of physician's assistant? (One response.)

Yes, I would accept either sex in the role of physician's assistant ____

No, regardless of the sex of the physician's assistant, I would not want to use the services of one ____

No, I would accept the physician's assistant only if he were a man ____

No, I would accept the physician's assistant only if she were a woman ____

(3) (A) Think about what the doctor does for you on each of your visits to his office. What parts (if any) of each visit would you be willing to have a trained physician's assistant do

for you as opposed to the doctor personally doing it for you? (You may check more than one.)

initial physical examination including the pelvic examination ____

initial physical examination excluding the pelvic examination ____

blood pressure ____

urine test ____

blood test ____

check baby's heartbeats ____

answer any questions about any problems I am having with my pregnancy ____

check baby's position and size such as the doctor does when he feels my abdomen ____

Other ____________
(Please be specific)

(B) What parts of your care during each visit would you be willing to have only the doctor do? (You may check more than one response.)

initial physical examination including the pelvic examination ____

initial physical examination excluding the pelvic examination ____

blood pressure ____

blood test ____

urine test ____

check baby's position and size ____

check baby's heartbeats ____

answer any questions about problems I am having during my pregnancy ____

(4) Would you be willing to have a trained physician's assistant deliver your baby? (Assume here that your doctor has previously checked you and determined that your delivery would be a normal one.)

Yes, only if the doctor is also present ____

Yes, the doctor need not actually be physically present ____

No ____

(5) If, by using the services of the physician's assistant, the total cost of your care during your pregnancy, labor, and delivery

were reduced, would you be more willing to use the services of the physician's assistant?

Yes _____

Yes, but it depends upon the amount of the decrease in the cost of care _____

No _____

(6) (A) Of the following people, which of them would you feel most comfortable with, and confident in, if this person were specially trained for the job of physician's assistant? (All of these people would have been exposed to the same additional training in order to qualify as a physician's assistant.) You may choose more than one response.

College graduate, with a health-related major (Ex. - Biology) _____

College graduate with a non-health-related major _____
Military Medic, recently discharged from the service _____
Registered Nurse, either male or female _____
Practical Nurse, either male or female _____
Hospital technician (Ex. - x-ray technician) _____
High School graduate _____
Junior College graduate _____
Any, if all were trained in a qualified physician's assistant training program _____

(B) Which one of the above categories of personnel would you prefer (only one) to be trained as a physician's assistant who would take care of you during your pregnancy?

____

(C) With reference to your answer to question no. 6B, why would you prefer this type of person to be educated as a physician's assistant? Why would you be more confident in this type of person as a physician's assistant? (Choose one response.)

already an accepted health worker _____

more educational preparation than others _____

has had more practical experience _____

I am used to this person working with the doctor already _____

Other _______________
(Please be specific)

(7) (A) What advantage (if any) do you see occurring if physician's assistants were used by your doctor? (You may check more than one answer.)

The doctor will be able to give more care to more patients ____

Cost of care may be reduced ____

There would be someone available (that is, the physician's assistant) to take more time to talk with me about my problems with the pregnancy than my doctor is usually able to do ____

Since the doctor will be less rushed with 'routine' care, the doctor would have more time to spend caring for particular problems I have during my pregnancy ____

Other ____________
(Please be specific)

(B) What of the advantages, which you mentioned above, would be most important to you in helping you to accept the care of a physician's assistant?

____

(8) (A) What disadvantages (if any) do you see occurring if physician's assistants were used by your doctor? (You may check more than one answer.)

I would get inferior care ____

I would be afraid the physician's assistant would not be able to tell if I had a problem until the problem had gotten very bad ____

I would not be able to discuss such personal problems with any one other than a real doctor ____

The doctor would be able to increase the number of patients he sees and then I would never get to see the doctor unless I had a very serious problem ____

Other ____________
(Please be specific)

(B) Which of the disadvantages, which you mentioned above (if any), would be most important to you in causing you to reject the care of a physician's assistant?

____

(9) (A) The use of the physician's assistant in an obstetrician's office may mean that the nurse will no longer be needed in your doctor's office. How do you feel about this? (Check only one answer.)

If it meant replacing the nurse in the obstetrician's office, I would not favor the use of the physician's assistant ____

I think the use of the physician's assistant in the obstetrician's office would probably replace the nurse in the office; however, this would be good for it would free the nurse to work in the hospital or other places where she may be more needed than in the obstetrician's office ____

I feel that there is a job for both the physician's assistant and the nurse in the obstetrician's office ____

(B) If you feel that there is a job for both the physician's assistant and the nurse in the obstetrician's office, how would you describe the job of the nurse as it differs from that of the physician's assistant?

(10) The physician's assistant may be hard for pregnant women to accept because of the special relationship between a pregnant woman and her doctor; however, if physician's assistants were used, what do you think would make you more comfortable about using them? (You may check more than one answer; however, place two checks by the answer which you feel would be most important to you in increasing your acceptance of the physician's assistant.)

If I know that they were adequately educated ____

If I knew that they would take the time to know me as a person ____

If my doctor hired the physician's assistant I know he would be a good one ____

Other ____________
(Please be specific)

(11) (A) Do you feel that there is a shortage of doctors to care for pregnant women in this community?

Yes ____ No ____

(B) Why do you feel there is a shortage of obstetricians here?

Had to wait a long time for an initial appointment ____

The doctor always seems so rushed ____

Other __________ Does not apply ____
(Please be specific)

(12) What have you found most disturbing about the care you are receiving from your obstetrician?

Doctors are always so rushed ____

Doctors do not seem to care about me as an individual ____

I see too many doctors; I do not really know any of them ____

Other __________
(Please be specific)

Nothing particularly disturbs me about the care I receive; I am satisfied with the care I get ____

(13) (A) Which of the following statements most closely fits your idea of what a doctor is? (Choose one response.)

To me, a doctor is a human 'miracle worker' ____

To me, a doctor is more than a healer of physical diseases; he is more of a friend - someone to whom I can speak about any personal problems about which I am worried ____

To me, a doctor is a highly educated professional who is able to help me with my health problems ____

To me, a doctor is an overpaid skilled technician ____

(B) In your own words, describe your feelings about a doctor; that is, what does 'an obstetrician' (not your own doctor) mean to you?

(14) Whom do you (did you) ask when you need advice about which obstetrician to go to?

friend ____ relative ____ nurse ____ family doctor ____

Other ____________
(Please be specific)

APPENDIX F

LIST OF NATIONAL PROGRAM RESPONDENTS: 1970 and 1973*

Early PA Programs:†

Child Health Associate Program
University of Colorado
Denver, Colorado

Clinical Associate Program
University of Kentucky
Lexington, Kentucky

Master Physician's Assistant in Anesthesiology Program
Emory University
Atlanta, Georgia

MEDEX Program
Dartmouth College
Hanover, New Hampshire

MEDEX Program
University of Washington
Seattle, Washington

Ophthalmic Assistant Program
Baylor University
Houston, Texas

Orthopaedic Assistant Program and Pediatrician's Assistant Program
Santa Clara County Medical Society
San Jose, California

Pathologist Assistant Program
University of Alabama
Birmingham, Alabama

Pediatric Assistant Program
Georgia State University
Atlanta, Georgia

Physician's Assistant Program
University of Florida
Gainesville, Florida

Physician's Assistant Program
Western Michigan University
Kalamazoo, Michigan

Physician's Assistant Program
Medical Center for Federal Prisoners
Springfield, Missouri

---

*Although the majority of the above programs participated in both the 1970 and 1973 surveys, a few programs responded to only one of the surveys. Several chose not to participate a second time and other programs had been discontinued in the interim period.

†This list is intended only as a means of identifying the PA programs participating in the surveys; therefore, the addresses are purposely incomplete. For an up-to-date list of PA programs, the reader is referred to the following governmental publication: Selected Training Programs for Physician Support Personnel, Division of Manpower Intelligence, U.S. Department of Health, Education, and Welfare (Washington, D.C., 1972).

Physician's Assistant Program
U.S. Public Health Service Hospital
Staten Island, New York

Physician's Assistant Program
Wake Forest University
Winston-Salem, North Carolina

Physician's Assistant Program
Cleveland Clinic Hospital
Cleveland, Ohio

Physician's Assistant Program
Alderson-Broaddus College
Philippi, West Virginia

Physician's Assistant Program
Marshfield Clinic
Marshfield, Wisconsin

Physician's Associate Program
Yale University
New Haven, Connecticut

Physician's Associate Program
Emory University
Atlanta, Georgia

Physician's Associate Program
Brooklyn-Cumberland Medical Center
Brooklyn, New York

Physician's Associate Program
Duke University
Durham, North Carolina

Physician's Associate Program
University of Oklahoma
Oklahoma City, Oklahoma

Surgeon's Assistant Program
University of Alabama
Birmingham, Alabama

Surgical Assistant Program
Massachusetts General Hospital
Boston, Massachusetts

Early NP Programs*

Family Nurse Practitioner Program
University of California, Davis
Davis, California

Medical Nurse Associate Program and Pediatric Nurse Associate Program
Presbyterian-St. Luke's Hospital
Chicago, Illinois

Nursing Pediatrist Program
U.C.L.A. School of Medicine
Torrance, California

Pediatric Nurse Associate Program
University of Maine
Portland, Maine

Pediatric Nurse Associate Program
Good Samaritan Hospital
Cincinnati, Ohio

---

*This list is intended only as a means of identifying the NP programs participating in the surveys; therefore, the addresses are purposely incomplete. For an up-to-date list of NP programs, the reader is referred to the following government publication: Preparing Registered Nurses for Expanded Roles: A Directory of Programs - 1973-74, Division of Manpower Intelligence, U.S. Department of Health, Education, and Welfare (Washington, D.C., 1974).

Pediatric Nurse Practitioner Program
Northeastern University
Boston, Massachusetts

Pediatric Nurse Practitioner Program
Washington University
St. Louis, Missouri

Pediatric Nurse Practitioner Program
University of Rochester
Rochester, New York

Pediatric Nurse Practitioner Program
St. Christopher's Hospital for Children
Philadelphia, Pennsylvania

Pediatric Nurse Practitioner Program
University of Washington
Seattle, Washington

Primary Health Care Nurse Practitioner Programs
University of Colorado
Denver, Colorado

BIBLIOGRAPHY

BOOKS AND REPORTS

Blum, Henrik L. Health Planning: 1969. San Francisco, California: American Public Health Association, 1970.

Coser, Lewis A. The Functions of Social Conflict. New York: The Free Press, 1956.

De Fleur, Melvin L., William V. D'Antonio, and Lois B. De Fleur. Sociology: Man in Society. Glenview, Ill.: Scott Foresman, 1971.

Fein, Rashi. The Doctor Shortage: An Economic Diagnosis. Washington, D. C.: The Brookings Institution, 1967.

Foster, George M. Traditional Cultures and the Impact of Technological Change. New York: Harper, 1962.

Ginzberg, Eli, with Miriam Ostow. Men, Money, and Medicine. New York: Columbia University Press, 1969.

Greenfield, Harry I., and Carol A. Brown. Allied Health Manpower: Trends and Prospects. New York: Columbia University Press, 1969.

Krause, Elliott A. The Sociology of Occupations. Boston: Little, Brown and Company, 1971.

Lionberger, Herbert F. Adoption of New Ideas and Practices. Ames, Iowa: The Iowa State University Press, 1960.

National Academy of Sciences. New Members of the Physician's Health Team's Physician's Assistants. Washington, D. C.: The Academy, 1970.

National Commission for the Study of Nursing and Nursing Education. An Abstract for Action. New York: McGraw-Hill, 1970.

_____ "Nurse Clinician and Physician's Assistant: The Relationship Between Two Emerging Practitioner Concepts." Rochester, New York: The Commission, 1971.

Pavalko, Ronald M. Sociology of Occupations and Professions. Itasca, Illinois: Peacock, 1971.

Rogers, Everett M., with F. Floyd Shoemaker. Diffusion of Innovations. New York: The Free Press, 1971.

Royal Commission on Medical Education 1965-68: Report. London: Her Majesty's Stationery Office, 1969.

Sadler, Alfred M., Blair L. Sadler, and Ann A. Bliss. The Physician's Assistant: Today and Tomorrow. New Haven: Yale University Press, 1972.

Sellitz, Claire, Marie Jahoda, Morton Deutsch, and Stuart Cook. Research Methods in Social Relations. 2d ed. New York: Henry Holt, 1960.

Siegel, Sidney. Nonparametric Statistics for the Behavioral Sciences. New York: McGraw-Hill, 1956.

Somers, Anne R. Health Care in Transition: Directions for the Future. Chicago: Hospital Research and Educational Trust, 1971.

U. S. Department of Health, Education, and Welfare. Preparing Registered Nurses for Expanded Roles: A Directory of Programs, 1973-74.

____ Selected Training Programs for Physician Support Personnel. Washington, D. C.: The Department, 1972.

ARTICLES

Adamson, T. Elaine. "Critical Issues in the Use of Physician Associates and Assistants." American Journal of Public Health 61, no. 9 (September 1971): 1765-1779.

"AHA Makes Statement on M. D. Assistants." American Journal of Nursing, March 1971, p. 438.

"AMA Unveils Surprise Plan to Convert R. N. into Medic." American Journal of Nursing 70, no. 4 (April 1970): 691, 724, 727.

American Medical Association. "Health Manpower Increases Set as Objective." American Medical News, November 2, 1970, p. 12.

____ Editorial. Journal of the American Medical Association 213, no. 11 (September 1970): 1765-1766.

American Medical Association. "Physician's Assistants: Considerable Interest - and Some Controversy." Journal of the American Medical Association 205, no. 12 (September 1968): 28.

American Medical Association's Committee on Nursing. "Medicine and Nursing in the 1970s: A Position Statement." Journal of the American Medical Association 213, no. 11 (September 1970): 1881-1883.

American Medical Association's Council on Health Manpower. "The Child Health Associate: A New Training Program in Colorado." Journal of the American Medical Association 212, no. 6 (May 1970): 1045-1046.

"American Nurses' Association Views the Emerging 'Physician's Assistant.'" International Nursing Review 19, no. 2 (1972): 190.

"Assistance for the Physician: Nurse Clinician or Physician Assistant." Occupational Health Nursing 19, no. 11 (November 1971): 28-29.

Ballenger, Martha D. "Legal Considerations: the Physician's Assistant." Hospitals: Journal of the American Hospital Association 45 (June 1971): 58-61.

Ballenger, Martha D., and E. Harvey Estes. "Licensure or Responsible Delegation?" New England Journal of Medicine 284, no. 6 (February 1971): 330-332.

Bates, Barbara. "Doctor and Nurse: Changing Roles and Relations." New England Journal of Medicine 283, no. 3 (July 1970): 129-134.

Bergman, Abraham B. "Physician's Assistants Belong in the Nursing Profession." American Journal of Nursing 71, no. 5 (May 1971): 975, 977.

Bergman, Abraham B., S. W. Dassel, and Ralph J. Wedgwood. "Time-motion Study of Practicing Pediatricians." Pediatrics 38 (August 1966): 254-263.

Bergman, Abraham B., Jeffrey L. Probstfield, and Ralph J. Wedgwood. "Task Identification in Pediatric Practice." American Journal of Diseases of Children 118 (September 1969): 459-468.

Bergen, Richard. "Irregular Assistants and Legal Risks." Journal of the American Medical Association 207, no. 6 (February 1969): 1231-1232.

Blamphin, John M. "Department of Defense may become a Major Supplier of Physicians' Assistants for the Civilian Health Field." Medical World News, December 11, 1970, p. 39.

Borland, Barry L., Franklin E. Williams, and David Taylor. "A Survey of Attitudes of Physicians on Proper Use of Physician's Assistants." Health Services Reports 87, no. 5 (May 1972): 467-472.

Breytspraak, Linda Marshall, and Louis R. Pondy. "Sociological Evaluation of the Physician's Assistant's Role Relations." Group Practice, March 1969, pp. 32-42.

Butter, Irene. "Health Manpower Research: A Survey." Inquiry 4, no. 4 (December 1967): 5-47.

Carlson, Clifford L., and Gary T. Athelstan. "The Physician's Assistant: Versions and Diversions of a Promising Concept." Journal of the American Medical Association 214, no. 10 (December 1970): 1855-1861.

Conant, Loring, et al. "Anticipated Patient Acceptance of New Nursing Roles and Physicians' Assistants." American Journal of Diseases of Children 122 (September 1971): 202-205.

"Concept of MD Assistant is Backed by NAS Board: Academy Group Endorses Plan, Urges Survey." Medical Tribune, 1970, pp. 10, 32.

Coye, Robert D., and Marc F. Hansen, "The 'Doctor's Assistant.'" Journal of the American Medical Association 209, no. 4 (July 1969): 529-533.

Creighton, H. "Changes in the Legal Aspects of Nursing." Hospital Progress, September 1971, pp. 87-94.

Curran, William J. "The California 'Physician's Assistants' Law." New England Journal of Medicine 283, no. 23 (December 1970): 1274-1275.

_____ "Legal Responsibility for Actions of Physicians' Assistants." New England Journal of Medicine 286, no. 5 (February 1972): 254.

_____ "New Paramedical Personnel - to License or Not to License?" New England Journal of Medicine 282, no. 19 (May 1970): 1085-1086.

Curran, William J. "'Physicians' Assistants': The Question of Legal Responsibility." American Journal of Public Health 60, no. 12 (December 1970): 2400-2401.

Darley, Ward, and Anne R. Somers. "Medicine, Money and Manpower - The Challenge to Professional Education: IV. New Training for New Needs." New England Journal of Medicine 276, no. 26 (June 1967): 1471-1478.

Dasco, Michael M. "Training of Allied Health Professionals and Physicians' Assistants." Bulletin of the New York Academy of Medicine 46, no. 12 (December 1970): 1107-1111.

Day, Lewis R., Rosemarie Egli, and Henry K. Silver. "Acceptance of Pediatric Nurse Practitioners." American Journal of Diseases of Children 119 (March 1970): 204-208.

Department of Health, Education, and Welfare Secretary's Committee to Study Extended Roles for Nurses. "Extending the Scope of Nursing Practice: A Report of the Secretary's Committee to Study Extended Roles for Nurses." Journal of the American Medical Association 220, no. 9 (May 1972): 1231-1236.

De Tornyay, Rheba. "Expanding the Nurse's Role Does Not Make Her a Physician's Assistant." American Journal of Nursing 71, no. 5 (May 1971): 974, 976.

Donovan, Joseph F. "A Medical Corpsmen Project." California Medicine 111, no. 6 (December 1969): 487-490.

Duke University. "Physician's Assistant Program: 1970-1971." Bulletin of Duke University 42, no. 6B (March 1970): 1-64.

_____"Physician's Associate Program: 1972-1973." Bulletin of Duke University 44, no. 9 (April 1972): 1-50.

Duncan, Burris, Ann N. Smith, and Henry K. Silver. "Comparison of the Physical Assessment of Children by Pediatric Nurse Practitioners and Pediatricians." American Journal of Public Health 61, no. 6 (June 1971): 1170-1176.

Egeberg, Roger O., and Leroy A. Pesch. "The Roles for Nurses." Journal of the American Medical Association 220, no. 9 (May 1972): 1237-1238.

Eichenberger, Ralph W., et al. "The Clinical Associate: Rationale for Training a New Health Professional." Journal of the Kentucky Medical Association, September 1969, pp. 677-680, 696.

Eichenberger, Ralph W., et al. "Kentucky Physicians' Response to a New Health Professional." Journal of the Kentucky Medical Association, May 1970, pp. 303-310.

Estes, E. Harvey. "The Critical Shortage - Physicians and Supporting Personnel." Annals of Internal Medicine 69, no. 5 (November 1968): 957-962.

____"The Duke Physician Assistant Program." Archives of Environmental Health 17 (November 1968): 690-691.

Estes, E. Harvey, and D. Robert Howard. "The Physician's Assistant in the University Center." Annals of the New York Academy of Sciences 166 (December 1969): 903-910.

Ewer, Robert W., et al. "The Clinical Associate: An Indiana Concept." Journal of the Indiana State Medical Association, March 1970, pp. 234-237.

Fein, Rashi. "An Economist's View: Medical Manpower - a Continuing Crisis." Journal of the American Medical Association 201, no. 11 (September 1967): 171-173.

Ford, Patricia Ann, S. Seacat Milvoy, and George A. Silver. "The Relative Roles of the Public Health Nurse and the Physician in Prenatal and Infant Supervision." American Journal of Public Health 56, no. 7 (July 1966): 1097-1103.

Fuchs, V.R. "Can the Traditional Practice of Medicine Survive." Archives of Internal Medicine 125 (1970): 154-156.

Goldstein, Joan. "Medical Corpsmen as a Source of Civilian Health Manpower for New Jersey." Medical Care 8, no. 3 (May-June 1970): 254-258.

"Government Programs Promote Training and Use of Physicians' Assistants." American Family Physician 3, no. 5 (May 1971): 163.

Gravenstein, J.S., J.E. Steinhaus, and P.P. Volpitto. "Analysis of Manpower in Anesthesiology." Anesthesiology 33, no. 3 (September 1970): 350-357.

Hanson, W. Lee. "An Appraisal of Physician Manpower Projections." Inquiry 7, no. 1 (March 1970): 102-113.

Haverty, J. Rhodes. "Distribution of Physicians Rendering Pediatric Care in Georgia." Journal of the Medical Association of Georgia, May 1970, pp. 169-172.

Hershey, Nathan. "An Alternative to Mandatory Licensure of Health Professionals." Hospital Progress, March 1969, pp. 71-74.

Hicks, Nancy. "Returning Medics No Longer Spurned as Civilian Health Aides." The New York Times, December 13, 1970.

Hiestand, Dale L. "Research into Manpower for Health Service." Milbank Memorial Fund Quarterly 44, no. 4 (October 1966): 146-181.

Howard, Robert B. "Adapting Medical Education to Meet Increasing Manpower Requirements: Medical Manpower - A Continuing Crisis." Journal of the American Medical Association 201, no. 11 (September 1967): 180-182.

Howard, D. Robert. "Development of the Physician's Assistant Concept - Duke University." Appalachia Medicine, September 1970, pp. 1-3.

Howard, D. Robert, and C. Emil Fasser. "Duke University's Physician's Assistant Program." Hospital Progress, February 1970, pp. 49-55.

Hudson, Charles L. "Expansion of Medical Professional Services with Nonprofessional Personnel." Journal of the American Medical Association 176, no. 10 (June 1961): 95-97.

Hughbanks, Janet, and Donald K. Freeborn. "Reivew of 22 Training Programs for Physician's Assistants 1969." HSMHA Health Reports 86, no. 10 (October 1971): 857-862.

Jacobi, Eileen M. "Officially Speaking..." RN 33, no. 10 (October 1970): 57, 82, 84.

Kadish, Joseph, and James W. Long. "The Training of Physician's Assistants: Status and Issues." Journal of the American Medical Association 212, no. 6 (May 1970): 1047-1051.

Kissick, William L. "Health Manpower in Transition." Milbank Memorial Fund Quarterly 46, no. 1 (January 1968): 53-90.

Lambertsen, Eleanor C. "Not Quite MD, More Than PA," Hospitals: Journal of the American Hospital Association 45 (December 1971): 70-76, 136.

Lave, Judith R., Lester B. Lave, and Thomas E. Morton. "The Physician's Assistant: Exploration of the Concept." Hospitals: Journal of the American Hospital Association 45 (June 1971): 42-51.

Leedham, Charles L. "Officially Speaking. . ." RN 33, no. 10 (October 1970): 88, 90.

Legal-Medicine Foundation. "The Physician's Assistant is Authorized in California." Professional Liability Newsletter 2, no. 7 (September 1970): 1-2.

_____ "The Standard of Care Issue and the Physician's Assistant." Professional Liability Newsletter 2, no. 7 (September 1970): 2-3.

Leininger, M.M., D.E. Little, and Doris Carnevali. "Primex." American Journal of Nursing 72, no. 7 (July 1972): 1274-1277.

Lewis, Charles E. "Acceptance of Physician's Assistants." Hospitals: Journal of the American Hospital Association 45 (June 1971): 62-64.

Litman, Theodor J. "Public Perceptions of the Physician's Assistant - A Survey of the Attitudes and Opinions of Rural Iowa and Minnesota Residents." American Journal of Public Health, March 1972, pp. 343-346.

McCormack, Regina C., Herbert M. Allen, and Eric L. Livers. "Family Doctors' Use of Office Assistants and Opinions Regarding Nurses in Primary Care." Southern Medical Journal 64, no. 4 (April 1971): 415-418.

McCormack, Regina C., and Charles W. Miller. "The Economic Feasibility of Rural Group Practice: Influence of Non-Physician Practitioners in Primary Care." Medical Care 10, no. 1 (January-February 1972): 73-80.

McGrath, John, Marjorie McKusick, and Bernadine Paulshock. "Need for Physicians' Assistants." Journal of the American Medical Association 214, no. 13 (October 1970): 147-148.

Minno, Frances P.F. "Unjustified Malpractice Fears are Preventing Use of Doctor's Assistants." Modern Hospital 116, no. 6 (June 1971): 71-72.

Myers, Hu C. "The Emerging Physician's Assistant." Maryland State Medical Journal 19 (September 1970): 68-72.

_____ "The Physician's Assistant in the Community Hospital and In Office Practice." Annals of the New York Academy of Sciences 166 (December 1969): 911-915.

"National Program for Certifying Physician's Assistants." Physician's Associate 3, no. 1 (January 1973): 22-24.

"One Doctor for 850 Persons." St. Petersburg Times, April 6, 1971: 1B, 10B.

Parker, Harry J., and John C. Delahunt. "Tasks for the Physician's Assistant: Reactions of Urban Physicians." Dallas Medical Journal, July 1972.

Patterson, Patricia K., and Abraham B. Bergman. "Time-motion Study of Six Pediatric Office Assistants." New England Journal of Medicine 281 (October 1969): 771-774.

Patterson, Patricia K., Abraham B. Bergman, and Ralph J. Wedgwood. "Parent Reaction to the Concept of Pediatric Assistants." Pediatrics 44, no. 1 (July 1969): 69-75.

"Physician's Assistant Exam is Readied." Medical World News, May 11, 1973, p. 72.

"The Physician's Assistant Programs." RN 33, no. 10 (October 1970): 43-46.

Pratt, Ralph D. "Determining Legal Sanction for the P.A." Physician's Associate 2, no. 2 (April 1972): 47-49.

Proger, S. "The Education of Different Types of Physicians for Different Types of Health Care." Pharos 35 (1972): 53-66.

Rosenstock, Irwin M. "Why People Use Health Services." The Milbank Memorial Fund Quarterly: Health Services Research I 44, no. 3, Part 2 (July 1966): 94-127.

Rosinski, E.F. "Education and the Role of the Physician." Journal of the American Medical Association 222 (1972): 473-475.

Schiff, Donald W., Charles H. Fraser, and Heather L. Walters. "The Pediatric Nurse Practitioner in the Office of Pediatricians in Private Practice." Pediatrics 44, no. 1 (July 1969): 62-68.

Shu, C.Y. "The Physician's Assistant." Hospitals: Journal of the American Hospital Association 45 (June 1971): 16, 23.

Silver, Henry K. "New Allied Health Professionals: Implications of the Colorado Child Health Associate Law." New England Journal of Medicine 284, no. 6 (February 1971): 304-307.

Silver, Henry K. "A New Primary-Care Medical Practitioner." American Journal of Diseases of Children 126 (September 1973): 324-327.

Silver, Henry, and Loretta Ford. "The Pediatric Nurse Practitioner at Colorado." American Journal of Nursing 67, no. 7 (July 1967): 1443-1444.

Silver, Henry K., and James A. Hecker. "The Child Health Associate." Hospitals: Journal of the American Hospital Association 44 (October 1970): 47-49.

Silver, Henry K., and John E. Ott. "The Child Health Associate: A New Health Professional to Provide Comprehensive Health Care to Children." Pediatrics 51, no. 1 (January 1973): 1-7.

Skinner, Alfred L. "Parental Acceptance of Delegated Pediatric Services." Pediatrics 41, no. 5 (May 1968): 1003-1004.

Stead, Eugene A. "Conserving Costly Talents - Providing Physicians New Assistants." Journal of the American Medical Association 198, no. 10 (December 1966): 182-183.

Theodore, Chris N. "Physician Support Personnel in the 70's - Economic Implications." Journal of the American Medical Association 214, no. 7 (November 1970): 1301-1302.

Todd, Malcolm C. "Medical Manpower and the Emergence of New Professions." Texas Medicine 68, no. 10 (October 1972): 60-64.

_____ "National Certification of Physicians' Assistants by Uniform Examinations." Journal of the American Medical Association 222, no. 5 (October 1972): 563-566.

Todd, Malcolm C., and Donald F. Foy. "Current Status of the Physician's Assistant and Related Issues." Journal of the American Medical Association 220, no. 13 (June 1972): 1714-1720.

Tucker, Murray. "Utilization and Price Analysis: Prospects for Avoiding Higher Program Costs in Health Care." American Journal of Public Health 209, no. 4 (July 1969): 529-533.

Walsh, Margaret E. "Officially Speaking..." RN 33, no. 10 (October 1970): 84, 86, 88.

Weiss, Jeffrey H. "A Job Classification Scheme for Health Manpower." Health Services Report 3, no. 1 (Spring 1968): 48-64.

Wolper, Lawrence F. "The Legal Status of the Physician's Assistant." Hospital Progress, October 1972, pp. 45-50, 67.

Yankauer, Alfred, et al. "The Outcomes and Service Impact of a Pediatric Nurse Practitioner Training Program - Nurse Practitioner Training Outcomes." American Journal of Public Health 62 (March 1972): 347-353.

____"The Practice of Nursing in Pediatric Offices - Challenge and Opportunity." New England Journal of Medicine 282 (April 1970): 843-847.

Yankauer, Alfred, John P. Connelly, and Jacob J. Feldman. "Physician Productivity in the Delivery of Ambulatory Care: Some Findings from a Survey of Pediatricians." Medical Care 8, no. 1 (January-February 1970): 35-46.

____"A Survey of Allied Health Worker Utilization in Pediatric Practice in Massachusetts and in the United States." Pediatrics 42, no. 5 (November 1968): 733-742.

____"Task Performance and Task Delegation in Pediatric Office Practice." American Journal of Public Health 59, no. 7 (July 1969): 1104-1117.

UNPUBLISHED MATERIALS

American Nurses' Association and American Academy of Pediatrics. "Guidelines on Short-Term Continuing Education Programs for Pediatric Nurse Associates." Mimeographed. New York: Division on Maternal and Child Health Nursing, American Nurses' Association, January 29, 1971.

Andrews, Priscilla M., and Yankauer, Alfred. "The Pediatric Nurse Practitioner at Work: Function, Role, and Identity." Mimeographed. Charlestown, Massachusetts: Pediatric Nurse Practitioner Program, Bunker Hill Health Center, December 1970.

Donovan, Joseph F. "Increasing Medical Manpower." Paper read before the meeting of the National Association of Blue Shield Plans, Chicago, Illinois, October 5-6, 1970. Mimeographed.

"Evaluation Report: Pediatric Nurse Associate Project." Mimeographed. Augusta, Maine: Regional Medical Program, January 1972.

Fry, Fred L. "A Study of the Acceptability of the Former Military Independent Duty Medical Corpsman as a Medical Resource in Rural Communities." Master's thesis, Oklahoma State University, May 1970. Mimeographed.

Gravenstein, J. S., Steinhaus, J. E., and Volpitto, P. P. "Three-University Study of Manpower in Anesthesia." Mimeographed. Atlanta, Georgia: Department of Anesthesiology, Emory University, 1970.

Henry, Richard A. "Professional Assistant and Associate in Medicine Program." Mimeographed. Program proposal. Gainesville, Florida: Division of Community Health, Department of Medicine, University of Florida, September 1970.

Hoekelman, Robert A. "The Pediatric Nurse Practitioner: An Analysis of Potential Training and Utilization in New York State. Mimeographed. Rochester, New York: Department of Pediatrics, University of Rochester, January 1971.

"Legislative Proposal for Physician's Assistants." Mimeographed. Durham, North Carolina: Department of Community Health Sciences, Duke University, October 1970.

"Marine Physician's Assistant Training Center: Curriculum." Mimeographed. Program brochure. Staten Island, New York: U. S. Public Health Service Hospital, July 1970.

"Model Legislation Project for Physician's Assistants." Mimeographed. Durham, North Carolina: Department of Community Health Sciences, Duke University, August 1972.

"Physician's Assistant Program: Alderson-Broaddus College." Mimeographed. Program brochure. Philippi, West Virginia: Alderson-Broaddus College, undated.

Pondy, Louis R., et al. "A Study of Patient Acceptance of the Physician's Assistant." Mimeographed. Durham, North Carolina: Department of Community Health Services, Duke University, February 1970.

Silver, Henry K. "The Pediatric Nurse Practitioner and the Child Health Associate: New Types of Health Professionals." Paper read before the seminar on "Education in the Health-Related Professions" of the New York Academy of Sciences, New York, March 28, 1969. Mimeographed.

"Surgeon's Assistant Training Program." Mimeographed. Program brochure. Birmingham, Alabama: Medical Center and School of Medicine, University of Alabama, undated.

Turner, Irene, et al. "Evaluation of the Nurse Associate in a Variety of Health Care Settings." Mimeographed. Chicago: Rush Presbyterian-St. Luke's Medical Center, September 1973.

Yankauer, Alfred, and Andrews, Priscilla M. "The Pediatric Nurse Practitioner at Work: A Review of Evaluative Studies." Mimeographed. Charlestown, Massachusetts: Pediatric Nurse Practitioner Program, Bunker Hill Health Center, December 1970.

CORRESPONDENCE

Brooklyn-Cumberland Medical Center. Letter from Mary N. Nettles, R. N., Instructor, Medical Services Associate Program, Brooklyn-Cumberland Medical Center, Brooklyn, New York. February 5, 1971.

Duke University Medical Center. Letter from D. Robert Howard, M. D., Director, Physician's Assistant Program, Duke University Medical Center, Durham, North Carolina. January 11, 1971.

Emory University. Letter from John E. Steinhaus, M. D., Professor and Chairman, Department of Anesthesiology, Emory University School of Medicine, Atlanta, Georgia. January 12, 1971.

Good Samaritan Hospital. Letter from Donald J. Frank, M. D., Director, Pediatric Nurse Associate Program, Good Samaritan Hospital, Cincinnati, Ohio. January, 1971.

Santa Clara County Medical Society. Letter from Joseph F. Donovan, Executive Director, Santa Clara County Medical Society, San Jose, California. March 11, 1971.

United States Public Health Service Hospital. Letter from James H. Hensley, M. P. H., Director of Training, Marine Physician Assistant Program, U.S. Public Health Service Hospital, Staten Island, New York. March 16, 1971.

University of Alabama. Letter from Margaret K. Kirklin, M. D., Director, Surgeon's Assistant Training Program, Department of Surgery, Medical Center, University of Alabama in Birmingham, Birmingham, Alabama. March 10, 1971.

University of California. Letter from Jean G. French, D. P. D., Director, Family Health Practitioner Program, School of Public Health, University of California, Berkeley, California. March 14, 1971.

University of Colorado. Letter from James A. Hecker, M. D., Associate Director, Child Health Associate Program, Medical Center, University of Colorado, Denver, Colorado. January 8, 1971.

Western Michigan University. Letter from George G. Mallinson, Dean and Chairman, Ad Hoc Committee on Physician's Assistants, The Graduate College, Western Michigan University, Kalamazoo, Michigan. January 29, 1971.

ABOUT THE AUTHOR

Ann Suter Ford is a Research Associate in Health Planning and a doctoral candidate in the Department of Urban and Regional Planning, The Florida State University, Tallahassee. In addition to five years of clinical nursing experience, she has worked as a health planner for both the Division of State Planning (formerly the Bureau of Planning) and the Bureau of Comprehensive Health Planning in the State of Florida. During these periods, she authored several in-house reports on health delivery problems in the family planning area, in the provision of health services to the medically indigent, and provided background information for the development of state legislation for health maintenance organizations. She is an Associate Member of the American Institute of Planners.

Mrs. Ford received her diploma in nursing in 1964 from the White Plains Hospital School of Nursing in White Plains, New York, her B.S.N. "with high distinction" from the University of Kentucky in 1967, and her M.S. in Urban and Regional Planning from The Florida State University in 1971. She is a member of the Phi Kappa Phi scholastic honorary society.

RELATED TITLES
Published by
Praeger Special Studies

AMERICAN HEALTH: Professional Privilege vs. Public Need
Tom Levin

HEALTH CARE TEAMS: An Annotated Bibliography
Monique K. Tichy

MANPOWER SUBSTITUTION IN THE HOSPITAL INDUSTRY: A Study of New York City Voluntary and Municipal Hospital Systems
Myron D. Fottler

THE NEW HUMAN SERVICE WORKER: Community College Education and the Social Services
Edward Allan Brawley

PARAPROFESSIONALS AND THEIR PERFORMANCE: A Survey of Education, Health, and Social Service Programs
Alan Gartner